HIV/AIDS
Problems, Causes and Control

HIV/AIDS

Problems, Causes and Control

A.K. YADAV

2007

CYBER TECH PUBLICATIONS

4264/3 Ansari Road, Daryaganj, New Delhi - 110 002

HIV/AIDS: Problems, Causes and Control

First Edition 2007

Published by G.S. Rawat
For Cyber Tech Publications
4264/3, Ansari Road, Daryaganj, New Delhi - 110 002
E-mail : cybertechpublishers@yahoo.com
Phone : 011-23244078,
Fax : 011-23280028

Printed at
Tanwar Offset Press, Moujpur, # 9810878184

Preface

The epidemic of HIV/AIDS, is largely looming all over the world. This is going to be more dangerous than atomic weapons. So far no remedy is available for cure; only can be prevented.

The Human Immunodeficiency Virus (HIV) basically provokes an infection, which destroys the body's immune system. And AIDS or Acquired Immune Deficiency Syndrome is the advanced stage of this disease, when the immune system becomes irreparably damaged, engendering multiple infections and cancers.

According to the recent estimates of UNAIDS around the world an estimated 40 million people are living with HIV/AIDS. 2.3 million of them children. Over the next decade without effective treatment and care, they will join the ranks of the more than 20 million people who have died of AIDS since the first clinical evidence of HIV/AIDS was reported in 1981. It is equally clear that the vast majority of people (including those living in countries with high national HIV prevalence) have not yet acquired the virus. Enabling them to protect themselves against HIV, and providing adequate and affordable treatment and care to people living with the virus, represent two of the biggest challenges facing humankind today.

HIV/AIDS marks a severe development crisis in almost all countries of the world, especially in sub-Saharan Africa, which remains by far the worst-affected region in the world.

Beyond sub-Saharan Africa, the epidemics of HIV/AIDS continue to grow in China, Indonesia, Papua New Guinea, Vietnam, many Central Asian Republics, the Baltic States, and North Africa. Vietnam, for example, provides fresh evidence of how an HIV/ AIDS epidemic can erupt suddenly wherever significant levels of injecting drug use occurs. It has joined a growing list of countries in Asia. Eastern Europe, the Middle East and Latin America, where injecting drug use has primed HIV/AIDS epidemics. In such settings, as in the epidemic generally, stigma and discrimination rank high among the obstacles that hinder efforts to turn the tide of AIDS.

This book consists of some select readings, mainly focussing on problems, causes and prevention of this dreaded disease. Substantially based on authoritative secondary sources, the vital information is contained under the following chapters, namely—Introduction; Vulnerable India; Fighting HIV: Some Guidelines; and Effective Counselling: Methods & Techniques. An exhaustive glossary of relevant terms and bibliography are added features.

Since the material is liberally drawn from various sources and research findings of many individuals and agencies working incessantly in the direction of HIV/AIDS at national/international level, we owe a deep sense of gratitude to them all, our aim being to disseminate the relevant information to readers, thus contribute to AIDS awareness.

We are equally grateful to persons/libraries, at the helm of affairs, for helping to make requisite information available. Finally, our publisher deserves all appreciation to bring out this book in nice getup within shortest possible time.

—DKL

Contents

CHAPTER 1

Introduction

Of late, no other word engenders as much fear, revulsion, despair and utter helpless AIDS. Despite increased AIDS awareness, the terror persists. AIDS is, in fact, rewriting medical history as humankind's deadliest scourge. With 40 million deaths forecast in this millennium, statistics tell their own sordid tale.

The first recorded sample of HIV was discovered in 1959 in a blood specimen obtained at Leopoldville (now Kinshasa) in the Belgian Congo. This was the first known death chalked up by AIDS.

The HIV is thought to have originally affected chimpanzees. The crossover of the virus from animals to humans may have occurred in the 1950s through an accident or a bite. Intermittently, other theories of its origins have been advanced during the ongoing process of AIDS research.

One theory, put forward by Bette Korber, traces the disease to a single viral ancestor that could have emerged between 1910 and 1950. Through an AIDS research analysis done at the Los Alamos National Lab in New Mexico, Korber contends that the pandemic may have come from one or more infected humans around 1930.

Remarkably, a highly controversial--but plausible--theory is that of American philosopher, Louis Pascal, first spelt out in 1987. All the early AIDS cases originated in the Central African states of Congo, Rwanda or Burundi. This belt was subjected to trials of a live polio vaccine on 300,000 men, women and children. Pascal argued that the vaccine, which was grown in cultures obtained from chopped up chimpanzee kidneys, may have carried this virus. Polio researcher Dr Albert Sabin had reported that such a batch was contaminated by an unknown virus. In fact, monkeys harbor SIV or simian immunodeficiency virus (SV-40 to be more specific), which is thought to be the ancestor of HIV.

The first cases of AIDS were reported in the United States in 1981, amongst male homosexuals in Los Angeles and New York. Within two decades, up to 50 million may have been infected globally, approximately 22 million have succumbed and nearly 15,000 new infections are said to occur daily. With a definite AIDS cure still in the research stages, an increased AIDS awareness, counseling and alternative therapy treatments seem to offer the only succor.

What is AIDS & HIV?

HIV has two major categories: HIV-1 and HIV-2. HIV-1, which currently has about 10 subtypes, is most common worldwide and the only form found in the US. HIV-2 is less virulent and though currently confined to West Africa--it's spreading. The Human Immunodeficiency Virus (HIV) basically provokes an infection, which destroys the body's immune system. And AIDS or Acquired Immune Deficiency Syndrome is the advanced stage of this disease, when the immune system becomes irreparably damaged, engendering multiple infections and cancers.

A person is considered HIV positive when s/he tests positive for any of the 26 diseases (Kaposi's sarcoma, lymphoma, pulmonary tuberculosis, recurrent pneumonia within a 12-month period, wasting syndrome and other indicators) that can easily invade body during our immune system's nonfunctionality.

On invading the body, the virus specifically attacks T-cells. A core part of the defence system, they mobilize other cells to seek and destroy contagious for elements besides leading the immune system's fight against infections. T-cell targeted because the AIDS virus parasitizes the CD4 molecules on their surface

With a protective outer shell of proteins and glycoproteins, the AIDS virus contains genetic information on the inside. Although substantially smaller than the host T-cells—the virus reproduces by sponging off the host's cellular resources Our fights back by producing up to two billion new T-cells to replace the infected stabilising the T-cell count temporarily. Yet from day one, the T-cells fight a battle.

The genetic information of the AIDS virus, which is encoded as RNA (ribonucleic acid), needs to be reverse transcripted--which the intruder accomplishes with the help of the host cell itself! The now legible DNA is thereafter randomly transferred into the nucleus. All this is accomplished barely a dozen hours following the infection. By this time, the aggressor begins to substantially weaken the host cell, which eventually dies, eroding the immune system and making the body vulnerable to diseases.

Although HIV targets T-cells and other cells in the body, it thrives mainly in the lymph nodes--another important part of the immune system. Each lymph node has a netlike structure inside it that acts as a protective filter by trapping virus and infected T-cells. But as healthy T-cells move through contaminated lymph nodes, they are infected by HIV. Particularly during the early stage of the disease, lymph nodes contain more infected cells than the blood.

Symptoms of Disease

In the early stages, a mild flu and swollen glands are typical. But the symptoms are often unmistakeable when full-blown AIDS develops. Loss of appetite, weight loss, constant fever, prolonged fatigue, diarrhea, constipation, changing bowel patterns, swollen glands, chills coupled with excessive sweating, especially at nights, lesions in the mouth, sore throat, persistent cough, shortness of breath, tumours, skin rashes, headaches, memory lapses, swelling in the joints, pain in various parts of the body, vision problems and a regular feeling of lethargy and ill health make up the litany of symptoms. With immune systems out of kilter, HIV-positive persons are susceptible to several types of cancer, particularly Kaposi's sarcoma (KS), an uncommon form that occurs under the skin and in the mucus membranes of the eyes, nose and mouth. Affected persons have lesions that appear as dark-coloured raised blotches. Though the lesions are painless, once KS spreads to the lungs, lymph nodes and digestive tract, the victim experiences difficulty in breathing, gastrointestinal bleeding and painful swelling around the lymph nodes, especially in the legs.

How HIV Transmits?

HIV is transmitted primarily by sex (anal, vaginal or oral sex with an infected partner), by injections (sharing contaminated needles for drug use or accidental piercing with a contaminated needle), or from infected mother to child through pregnancy or breast-feeding.

Infected semen and vaginal fluids, infected blood and blood products lead to the transmission of HIV. Drug abuse with unsterilised needles is another high-risk activity. Unprotected sex with multiple partners is the primary cause of infection. During unprotected sex, the infected fluid could enter the bloodstream through a tiny cut or a sore.

Anal penetration has a higher risk of transmission, which is why a high percentage of homosexuals develop the disease. Bleeding during sex also raises the chances of infection. Therefore unprotected sex during menstrual periods and anal intercourse are best avoided. An infected mother can also transmit the virus to her baby before or during birth or through breast milk. Although traces of HIV have been detected in body fluids (saliva, urine, faeces and tears) there is no evidence that HIV spreads through these fluids. Nor is it water-borne, air-borne or transmitted through mosquitoes and other insects.

Some HIV-infected patients progress to AIDS quickly while others can remain healthy for 10 years or more. Between initial infection and full-blown disease, a middle phase called symptomatic HIV infection, or AIDS-related complex (ARC), occurs, prompting symptoms such as weight loss, diarrhea, and swollen lymph glands.

Scientists have recently discovered clues to why some patients develop AIDS quickly. In a study published in the journal *Science,* National Cancer Institute researchers found that inherited genes may set the clock for AIDS progression. Certain gene patterns tend to stave off AIDS, while others promote it. The researchers say the study may help lead to an AIDS-preventive vaccine or improved therapies against the virus.

HIV risk factors among injection drug users (IDUs) differ markedly by gender, according to a 10-year study funded by the National Institute on Drug Abuse (NIDA). A recent study by researchers at the Johns Hopkins University reported that while drug-related risk behaviors and homosexual activity are the most important predictors of HIV seroconversion among males, factors consistent with high-risk heterosexual activities are the main predictors among females.

"Early studies of injection drug users suggested that most HIV infections were due primarily to sharing needles," said NIDA Director Alan I. Leshner, Ph.D. "This study adds to the body of evidence that supports the need for gender-specific interventions in the treatment of that group of drug users."

Between 1988 and 1998, a team of researchers, led by Dr. Steffanie Strathdee at the Johns Hopkins University Bloomberg School of Public Health, examined both drug related and sexual risk factors for HIV transmission in a study of more than 1,800 injecting drug users in Baltimore, Maryland. Study participants were aged 18 or older, did not have an AIDS defining illness at enrollment, and reported a history of illicit injection drug use within the previous 10 years. Through semiannual interviews, researchers collected data on drug use history, sociodemographics, and drug use and sexual behavior within the last 6 months. Blood samples were also obtained at each study visit. Researchers used commercial HIV and antibody ELISA to identify those participants who had become HIV positive since their last visit.

Dr. Strathdee and her colleagues found that the greatest predictor for HIV seroconversion among both male and female IDUs was high-risk sexual behavior. Study findings revealed that male injection drug users who reported recent homosexual activity were four times more likely to become infected with HIV.

Among females, indicators of high-risk heterosexual activity outweighed needle-sharing behaviors as independent predictors of HIV seroconversion. HIV incidence was more than two times higher among women who reported recently having sex with another injection drug user.

Another common predictor of HIV seroconversion observed by researchers among both male and female IDUs was younger age. Investigators found that IDUs who were aged 30 or younger at enrollment were more than twice as likely to seroconvert than those aged 40 or older.

Prevention

While AIDS is a high-risk disease it can be prevented if proper precautions are taken and greater awareness meted out to those who are ignorant of the virus and its repercussions on the human body. Here we have listed a few measures which can be adopted by everyone in order to stave off the insidious entry of HIV.

- Avoid intoxicants like, alcohol or drugs during sex, you might lose control of your senses and engage in unsafe sex. Stick to safer sex practices at all times and avoid having multiple partners. Practice monogamy. If this is a tall order, serial relationships are a lesser evil than multiple ones.

- Prevention is still the best bet. Promiscuous sexual behavior can leave a person highly susceptible to contracting the virus. Where abstinence is not possible, always use latex condoms. The female condom can also help protect both partners. Use only water-based lubricants. Oil lubricants (such as Vaseline) might even tear latex condoms. Use spermicidal (birth control) foams and jellies in addition to condoms. By themselves, spermicides may not be effective in preventing HIV.
- High-risk sexual behavior should be avoided at all costs.
- The presence of sexually transmitted diseases (STDs) increases the risk of contracting HIV from an infected partner. STDs could cause breaks in the skin of the vagina, penis or anus permitting the virus to enter your bloodstream. If you ever contract an STD of any kind, ensure you get prompt treatment.
- The CDC recommends that an HIV-positive woman should not breast-feed her baby. The infant should be given AZT for the first several weeks to substantially reduce the risk of infection.

Myths & Facts

Say 'AIDS' and dime-a-dozen misconceptions abound. The chart topper is that AIDS is supposedly a disease of gay men and intravenous drug users. The facts are otherwise. No doubt in the early years many HIV-positive cases were reported amongst the Western gay community. In recent years, however, prevalence rates among gays have leveled off. Instead, heterosexual transmission has been forging ahead of all other modes of transmission.

The AIDS virus is NOT contracted through touching, hugging, kissing, massage, sharing toilet seats, drinking or eating from utensils used by an infected person or any other mode of casual contact. Nor does working, socialising and living with infected people cause the disease.

Repeated sexual contact without proper precautions with an infected person, using an infected syringe, exposure to infected blood or sexual fluids are ways through which the disease can be transmitted. Donating blood also does not run the risk of disease contraction since needles used for such purposes are always sterile. Since the AIDS virus is unable to survive outside the human body beyond a short duration, dried blood is not infectious For this reason, mosquitoes are incapable of transmitting HIV as the virus cannot replicate itself in the intestine of insects.

Although medical personnel are potentially at risk from infection, this is minimal if protective gear such as gloves, masks and goggles are always used when handling potentially infected material.

The large-scale infections and deaths have spurred a spate of worldwide efforts for a cure. In the US, however, AIDS cases are said to be dropping and new infections leveling off. Mortality from AIDS is also dropping.

In the developing countries, though, the cases continue to rise alarmingly. Globally, three million died in the year 2000, with 5.3 million newly infected people, 95 per cent of whom might die. Many scientists, doctors and researchers contend that AIDS is not a new disease, having been around much longer than people believe.

Dr. Robert Willner--author of *Deadly Deception: The Proof That Sex and HIV Absolutely Do Not Cause AIDS*--

asserts that HIV is not the cause of AIDS. He claims that nearly 500 hundred top scientists of the world have challenged the hypothesis of Robert Gallo--who patented the HIV test the day after the AIDS virus was discovered--that HIV is the precursor of AIDS.

Dr. Frank Shallenberger, a licensed medical and homeopathic practitioner, says that statistics are only a correlation--not a result--that HIV is one cause of AIDS, citing the fact that some AIDS victims do not have HIV antibodies. Dr. Shallenberger considers AIDS a multifactorial disease that strikes when the immune system is down. The search for a cure, also brings to light other interesting facets. African chimpanzees have been harboring the simian equivalent of the AIDS virus for centuries, according to detailed studies conducted by researches at the University of Alabama in Birmingham. Why don't the chimps succumb to the virus? Says Dr. Anthony Fauci from the National Institute of Health: "There must be something about the chimp's immune system or some host defense system that is doing a very good job of containing the virus. If we find that out we may be able to extrapolate to humans."

Chimpanzees being the closest living relatives of humans, their DNA differs from human DNA by less than two per cent. Adds Dr. Fauci: "It's entirely conceivable that the very small genetic differences between the chimp and the human will explain why the chimpanzee does not get sick and the human does."

HIV (Human Immunodeficiency Virus) is a virus that causes AIDS (Acquired Immunodeficiency Syndrome), a health condition in which a person is affected by a series of diseases because of poor immunity. HIV by itself is not an illness and does not instantly lead to AIDS. An HIV infected person can lead a healthy life for several years before one develops AIDS.

As the name, Acquired Immunodeficiency Syndrome indicates, AIDS is a health condition that results from the deficiency in the body's immunity following HIV infection. HIV attacks the human body by breaking down its immune system that is meant to fight diseases. Over a period of time, the immune system weakens and the body loses its natural ability to fight diseases At this stage, various diseases affect the infected person.

Indian Scenario

India has among the highest number of persons living with HIV/AIDS in the world today, although the overall prevalence remains low. Some states experience a generalised epidemic with the virus transmitted from high-risk groups into the general population. A major challenge is to strengthen and decentralize the program to the state and district levels to enhance commitment, coverage and effectiveness.

State of the Epidemic

There are more than 5.1 million individuals infected with HIV in this country of over 1 billion people (UNAIDS 2003). The total number of AIDS cases in 2002 was estimated to be about 550,000. Seven states -- Andhra Pradesh, Goa, Karnataka, Maharashtra, Manipur, Mizoram, and Nagaland -- already have generalised epidemics, as indicated by a 1 per cent or higher prevalence rate among pregnant women in prenatal clinics. These seven states represent 22 per cent of the population.

Risk and Vulnerability

Several factors put India in danger of experiencing a rapid spread if effective prevention and control measures are not scaled up and expanded throughout the country. These risk factors include:

Unsafe Sex and Low Condom Use: In India, sexual transmission is responsible for 84 per cent of reported AIDS cases. HIV-prevalence rates are highest among sex workers and their clients, injecting drug users, and men who have sex with men (many of whom are married). When surveyed, 70 per cent of commercial sex workers in India reported that their main reason for not using of condoms was because their customers objected.

Migration and Mobility: Migration for work for extended periods of time takes migrants away from the social environment provided by their families and community. This can place them outside the usual normative constraints and thus more likely to engage in risky behavior. Concerted efforts are needed to address the vulnerabilities of the large migrant population.

Injecting Drug Use (IDU): Studies indicate that many drug users are switching from inhaling to injecting drugs. This phenomenon is more localised in the Northeastern states of India, and injecting drug users show sharp increases in HIV prevalence. Forty-one per cent of IDUs in a national survey reported injecting with used needles or syringes. Of those who cleaned their needles and syringes, only three per cent used an effective method such as alcohol, bleach, or boiling water. Appropriate strategies are also needed to address the double impact of drug use and unsafe sexual practices.

Low Status of Women: Infection rates have been on the increase among women and infants in some states. As in many other countries, unequal power relations and the low status of women, as expressed by limited access to human, financial, and economic assets, weakens the ability of women to protect themselves and negotiate safer sex, thereby increasing vulnerability.

Widespread Stigma: Stigma towards people infected with HIV/AIDS is widespread. The misconception that AIDS only affects men who have sex with men, sex workers, and injecting drug users strengthens and perpetuates existing discrimination. The most affected groups, often marginalised, have little or no access to legal protection of their basic human rights. Addressing the issue of human rights violations and creating an enabling environment that increases knowledge and encourages behavior change are thus extremely important to the fight against AIDS.

National Response to HIV/AIDS

Government: Shortly after reporting the first AIDS case in 1986, the Government of India established a National AIDS Control Program (NACP) which was managed by a small unit within the Ministry of Health and Family Welfare. The program's principal activity was then limited to monitoring HIV infection rates among risk populations in select urban areas.

In 1991, the strategy was revised to focus on blood safety, prevention among high-risk populations, raising awareness in the general population, and improving surveillance. A semi-autonomous body, the National AIDS Control Organisation (NACO), was established under the Ministry of Health and Family Welfare to implement this program. This "first phase" of the National AIDS Control Program lasted from 1992-1999. It focused on initiating a national commitment, increasing awareness and addressing blood safety.

It achieved some of its objectives, notably an increased

awareness. Professional blood donations were banned by law. Screening of donated blood became almost universal by the end of this phase. However, performance across states remained variable. By 1999, the program had also established a decentralised mechanism to facilitate effective state-level responses, although substantial variation continued to exist in the level of commitment and capacity among states. Whereas states such as Tamil Nadu, Andhra Pradesh, and Manipur demonstrated a strong response and high level of political commitment, many other states, such as Bihar and Uttar Pradesh, have yet to reach these levels.

The second phase of the NACP began in 1999 and will run until March 2006. Under this phase, India continues to expand the program at the state level. Greater emphasis has been placed on targeted interventions for high-risk groups, preventive interventions among the general population, and involvement of NGOs and other sectors and line departments, such as education, transport and police. Capacity and accountability at the state level continues to be a major issue and has required sustained support. Interventions need to be scaled up to cover a higher percentage of the population, and monitoring and evaluation need further strengthening. The Government has done away with the classification of states based on prevalence to avoid inducing complacency among states categorised as low prevalence, and has since focused on the vulnerability of states, hence creating a sense of urgency.

In brief, while the government's response has scaled up markedly over the last decade, major challenges remain in raising the overall effectiveness of state-level programs, expanding the participation of other sectors, and increasing safe behavior and reducing stigma associated with HIV-positive people among the population. The Government of India is currently in the early stages of preparing for the third phase of the National AIDS Control Program (NACP 3), for which a multi-disciplinary design team has been constituted to lead the preparation. The design of NACP 3 envisages a complex consultative process including nationwide consultations with various national stakeholders, as well as international development partners.

Role of NGOs

There are numerous NGOs working on HIV/AIDS issues in India at the local, state, and national levels. Projects include targeted interventions with high risk groups; direct care of people living with HIV/AIDS; general awareness campaigns; and care for AIDS orphans. Funding for NGOs comes from a variety of sources: the federal or state governments of India, international donors, and local contributions.

Notably, India receives technical assistance and funding from a variety of UN partners and bilateral donors. Bilateral donors such as USAID, CIDA, and DFID have been involved since the early 1990s at the state level in a number of states. USAID has committed more than US$70 million since 1992, CIDA US$ 11 million, and DFID close to US$200 million. The number of major financers and the amount of funding available has increased significantly in the last year. Since 2004, the Gates Foundation has pledged US$200 million for the next five years, the Global Fund has approved US$26 million for Prevention of Mother-to-Child Transmission (PMTCT) and about US$7 million for TB/HIV co-infection, and is considering another round of proposals, and USAID is considering the inclusion of India as its 15th priority country. DFID has also increased its financing and is considering the inclusion of additional states. Other more recent donors include DANIDA, SIDA, the Clinton Foundation and the European Union.

Issues and Challenges: Priority Areas

Limited Overall Capacity: There are severe institutional capacity constraints, including managerial, at the national and state levels. These are critical factors to address as the program attempts to scale-up the national response. NACO will require a change in its role and responsibilities to provide the necessary leadership and steering role for a stronger multisector response for the next phase in India's fight against HIV/AIDS.

Institutional arrangements and personnel turnover: There is a high turnover of state level project directors, resulting in limited continuity and variability in performance across states. This puts program growth at risk.

Use of Data for Decision Making: There remains a need for greater use of data for decision making, including program data and epidemiological data. A lot of data that is being generated is not adequately used for managing the program or inform policies and priorities. Results-based management and linking incentives to the use of data should be explored.

Donor Coordination: At present there are over 32 donor agencies working with NACO in different states and on different programs. Each donor comes with its own mandate and requirements, as well as areas of focus. The transaction cost to the government as a result of attending to the various demands of the donors is huge. There is a need for better coordinating mechanisms among the donors and clear leadership by the Government to reduce the transaction costs.

Variable Ability to Implement Responses Across States: The capacity to mount a strong program is weakest in some of the poorest and most populated states with significant vulnerability to the epidemic. There is a need for tailored capacity-building activities and the introduction of some performance-based financing approaches.

Stigma and Discrimination: Stigma and discrimination against people living with HIV/AIDS and those considered to be at high risk remain entrenched. A lot of this is a result of inadequate knowledge. For instance, more than 75 per cent of Indians mistakenly believed they could contract HIV from sharing a meal with a person who has the disease, according to a recent study. Stigma and denial undermine efforts to increase the coverage of effective interventions among high risk groups such as men having sex with men, commercial sex workers and injecting drug users. Harassment by police and ostracism by family and community drives the epidemic underground and decreases the reach and effectiveness of prevention efforts. Though there is significant increase in awareness, due to efforts by the government, there is much room for improvement.

Low Awareness in Rural Areas: Sentinel site behavioral surveillance, completed in 2001, showed high HIV/AIDS basic awareness levels (82.4 per cent in males and 70 per cent in females). However, rural women demonstrated very low rates of awareness in Bihar (21.5 percent), Gujarat (25 percent), and Uttar Pradesh (27.6 percent). New approaches need to be tried to reach rural communities with information about HIV/AIDS, safe sex and how to prevent and treat HIV/AIDS.

World Bank Response

In 1991, the Government of India and the World Bank

expanded their collaboration on infectious disease control programs and by 1992 the first National AIDS Control Project was launched with a World Bank credit of US$84 million. The project helped the government to broaden prevention efforts and to establish institutions and procedures necessary to curb the spread of HIV/AIDS. Building upon lessons learned from the first project, India requested World Bank financing for a follow-on project. With a World Bank credit of US$191 million, the Second National HIV/AIDS Control Project was started and this is increasing the pace of implementation through the use of State AIDS Societies to speed the distribution of funds at the state level.

The Bank has also undertaken analytical work to strengthen the national response, including an analysis of the full array of costs and consequences likely to result from several plausible government policy options regarding funding for anti-retroviral therapy (ART). Currently, the Bank is carrying out sector work on the economic consequences of the HIV/AIDS epidemic on India and is actively supporting the design of the third National AIDS Control Program.

Which AIDS Virus is Common in India?

The virus isolated from six individuals in India has been sequenced. Five turn out to be of type C (prevelant in Asia) and one a mosaic of types A and C. AIDS treatments developed against the type B virus prevelant in the US may be less effective in India.

Vulnerability

Perhaps 3 to 5 million people in India are living with HIV (in 1997). Infection rates nationally are less than 1%, although high-risk groups, specially in big cities, may have over 50% infection rates.

The incidence of HIV in Mumbai has grown rapidly since the first surveys were performed in 1989. Random testing of different segments of the population show different levels of incidence. Alarmingly large incidence rates of 51% have been found among sex-workers in Mumbai. Spread into the general hetero-sexual population has been found in a random testing of pregnant women in Mumbai which showed incidence rates of 2.4% (in 1996). Similar rates were found among blood donors in various government run hospitals.

To sum up, Overall, the incidence rate in India is about 0.7%, of which an alarmingly high 16.6% is due to infected blood, unclean syringes and other medical inefficiencies. In Maharashtra, the incidence climbs to 1.14%, which is close to twice the national average.

Ways to Control

The central government has set up the *National AIDS Control Organisation* as a nodel organisation to formulate policy and implement programs for the control of HIV/AIDS in India.

A sustained awareness campaign among the high-risk population of the *sex workers in Kamathipura* has yielded some benefits. However, institutional safeguards for blood banks and other health care units still leave a lot of scope for improvement.

The state government of Maharashtra has drawn up an *official HIV/AIDS control program,* and has received Rs. 21 crores (210 million) out of a Rs. 220 crore (2.2 billion) loan from the *World Bank.*

II

GLOBAL TRENDS

According to the recent estimates of UNAIDS around the world an estimated 40 million people are living with HIV/ AIDS. 2.3 million of them children. Over the next decade without effective treatment and care, they will join the ranks of the more than 20 million people who have died of AIDS since the first clinical evidence of HIV/AIDS was reported in 1981. It is equally clear that the vast majority of people (including those living in countries with high national HIV prevalence) have not yet acquired the virus. Enabling them to protect themselves against HIV, and providing adequate and affordable treatment and care to people living with the virus, represent two of the biggest challenges facing humankind today.

TABLE 1

Global summary of the HIV/AIDS epidemic (December 2003)

Number of people living with HIV /AIDS	
Total	40 million (34 - 16 million
Adults	37 million (31 -43 million)
Children under 15 years	2.5 million (2.1 - 2.9 million)
People newly infected with HIV in 2003	
Total	5 million (4.2 - 5.8 million)
Adults	4.2 million (3.6 -4.8 million)
Children under 15 years	700.000 (590 000 - 810.000)
AIDS deaths in 2003	
Total	3 million (2.5 - 3.5 million)
Adults	2.5 million (2.1 - 2.9 million)
Children under 15 years	500.000 (420 000 - 580.000)

REGIONAL TRENDS

HIV/AIDS marks a severe development crisis in almost all countries of the world, especially in sub-Saharan Africa, which remains by far the worst-affected region in the world. Beyond sub-Saharan Africa, the epidemics of HIV/AIDS continue to grow in China, Indonesia, Papua New Guinea, Vietnam, many Central Asian Republics, the Baltic States, and North Africa. Vietnam, for example, provides fresh evidence of how an HIV/ AIDS epidemic can erupt suddenly wherever significant levels of injecting drug use occurs. It has joined a growing list of countries in Asia. Eastern Europe, the Middle East and Latin America, where injecting drug use has primed HIV/AIDS epidemics. In such settings, as in the epidemic generally, stigma and discrimination rank high among the obstacles that hinder efforts to turn the tide of AIDS.

Sub-Saharan Africa

Sub-Saharan Africa remains by far the region worst-affected by the HIV/AIDS epidemic. In 2003, an estimated 26.6 million people in this region were living with HIV, including the 3.2 million who became infected during the past year. AIDS killed approximately 2.3 million people in 2003. Unlike women in other regions in the world, African women are considerably more likely--at least 1.2 times--to be infected with HIV than men. Among young people aged 15-24. this ratio is the highest: women were found to be two-and-a-half times as likely to be HIV-infected as their male counterparts, according to six recent national surveys. These discrepancies have been attributed to several factors. They include the biological fact that HIV generally is more easily transmitted from men to women (than vice versa). As well, sexual activity tends to start earlier for women, and young women tend to have sex with much older partners.

HIV prevalence varies considerably across the continent--ranging from less than 1 per cent in Mauritania to almost 40 per cent in Botswana and Swaziland. More than one in five pregnant women are HIV-infected in most countries in Southern Africa, while elsewhere in sub-Saharan Africa median HIV prevalence in antenatal clinics exceeded 10 per cent in a few countries. And while sustained prevention efforts in a few countries in West and East Africa continue to demonstrate that HIV/AIDS can he checked with human intervention. signs that similar inroads might be building in Southern Africa remain tenuous, at best.

Eastern Europe and Central Asia

The AIDS epidemic in Eastern Europe and Central Asia shows no signs of abating. Some 230,000 people were infected with HIV in 2003. bringing the total number of people living with the virus to 1.5 million. AIDS claimed an estimated 30,000 lives in the past year. The worst-affected are the Russian Federation Ukraine, and the Baltic States (Estonia, Latvia and Lithuania) but HIV continues to spread in Belarus. Moldova and Kazakhstan, while more recent epidemics are now evident in Kyrgyzstan and Uzbekistan. HIV prevalence continues to rise in the Russian Federation, which remains saddled with the worst epidemic in this region. By the end of 2002, a cumulative total of 229,000 people had been diagnosed with HIV. Almost a quarter of that total was added in 2002 alone, indicating that the epidemic is growing at a fearsome rate. Moreover, these reported cases almost certainly grossly underestimate the number of people living with HIV.

Asia and the Pacific

Over 1 million people in Asia and the Pacific acquired HIV in 2003, bringing to an estimated 7.4 million the number of people now living with the virus. A further

500.000 people are estimated to have died of AIDS in 2003. National adult HIV prevalence is still under 1 per cent in the majority of this region's countries. Several countries in the region are so large and populous that national aggregations can obscure serious epidemics in some provinces and states.

The HIV/AIDS picture in South Asia remains dominated by the epidemic in India, where between 3.82 and 4.58 million people were infected nationally by the end of 2002. In neighbouring Bangladesh and Nepal, national HIV prevalence has remained under 1 per cent, but risky behaviour in parts of the population is so extensive that it could be just a matter of time before wider epidemics erupt. In the Nepalese capital. Kathmandu. HIV epidemics are centred around injecting drug users and sex workers, most of them young. Among the former, HIV prevalence of up to 68 per cent has been detected recent years, while, among the latter, prevalence is around 17 per cent.

Latin America and the Caribbeans

Unfortunately, over 2 million people are now living with HIV in Latin America and the Caribbeans, including the estimated 200.000 that contracted HIV in the past year. At least 100.000 people died of AIDS in the same period--the highest regional death toll after sub-Saharan Africa and Asia. HIV/AIDS is well entrenched in this region, with national HIV prevalence at least 1 per cent in 12 countries, all of them in the Caribbean Basin. The most recent national estimates showed HIV prevalence among pregnant women reaching or exceeding 2 per cent in six of them the Bahamas, Belize, the-Dominican Republic, Guyana. Haiti, and Trinidad and Tobago. In contrast, most of the other countries of the region have highly concentrated epidemics. notably in South America where Brazil is home to the vast majority of people living with HIV in the region. Two of the region's most serious epidemics are on Hispaniola Island—in Haiti and the Dominican Republic. Stricken with the lowest health and other development indicators in the entire region. Haitians' woes are being aggravated dramatically by the AIDS epidemic, which is claiming an estimated 30,000 lives a year and has left some 200,000 children orphaned by AIDS. Haiti's national HIV prevalence levels have remained at 5-6 per cent since the late 1980s. The factors contributing to this apparent levelling off of national HIV prevalence are unclear, although it must be noted that sentinel surveillance has shown that HIV prevalence levels vary dramatically. With about 60 per cent of the population under 24 years of age, much scope exists for renewed growth in Haiti's mainly hetero-sexually transmitted epidemic. Condom use is very low among young people, despite evidence that HIV/AIDS knowledge is comparatively strong.

Middle East and North Africa

The notion that this region has sidestepped the global HIV epidemic is not borne out by the latest estimates, which indicate that 55,000 people acquired HIV infection in the year 2002 bringing to 600,000 the total number of people living with HIV/ AIDS in the Middle East and North Africa. AIDS killed a further 45,000 people in 2003. There is the potential for a considerable rise in the number of HIV infections in this region. By far the most seriously affected country at present is the Sudan--specifically the south, where a mainly heterosexual epidemic is well under way. Available data indicate a national adult HIV prevalence of more than 2 per cent, but conflict is hampering both surveillance of the epidemic and the mounting of a potentially effective response. The last round of surveillance data showed that HIV prevalence among pregnant women was six to eight times higher in the south of Sudan. Compared to Khartoum. HIV spread in this region appears to be nascent, although scant surveillance data in several countries could mean that serious outbreaks in certain populations may be being missed. There also appears to be significant movement of HIV-infected persons between some countries. More than half of those officially reported to have HIV in Tunisia, for example, are believed to have crossed the border from Libya to seek anti-retroviral treatment and/or to undergo drug rehabilitation. The epidemic threatens to expand along diverse routes in the region, including through blood transfusions and blood collection.

Universal precautions and blood screening have greatly reduced the risks of transmission in health-care settings in most countries, but HIV transmission through blood and blood products remains a potentially significant danger in somc. Also of concern is the rise in HIV infections among injecting drug users, particularly in Bahrain. Libya and Iran, while HIV infections linked to this mode of transmission have been reported in Algeria, Egypt, Kuwait, Morocco, Oman and Tunisia.

High-income Countries

The total number of people living with HIV continues to rise in high-income countries, largely due to widespread access to anti-retroviral treatment. It is estimated that 1.6 million people are living with HIV in these countries--a figure includes the 80.000 who were newly infected in 2003. AIDS claimed approximately 18.000 lives in the past year. The number of annual AIDS deaths has continued to slow in high-income countries, including those in Western Europe, due to the widespread availability of anti-retroviral treatment. There is mounting evidence that prevention activities in several high-income countries are not keeping pace with the changes occurring in the spread of HIV. Such shortcomings are most evident where HIV is lodged also among marginalised sections of populations, including immigrants and refugees.

In the United States of America, around half of the approximately 40,000 new infections annually are occurring among African-Americans (12 per cent .of the country's population), with African-American women accounting for an increasing proportion of new infections. Many of the women do not engage in high-risk behaviour, but are contracting HIV through unsafe sex with their male partners--a significant share of whom also have sex with men or inject drugs. Analysing data from 11 States, a recent US Centers for Disease Control and Prevention study found that 34 per cent of HIV, positive African-American men said they had sex with both women and men. However, only a small proportion of HIV positive African-American women reported knowing that their partner's also had sex with men. The secrecy surrounding such overlapping risk behaviour seems rooted mainly in the stigma that remains attached to homosexuality. The costs are steep: AIDS is now the leading cause of death for African-American women aged 25-34. According to the Centres for Disease Control, some 90 per cent of young urban HIV-positive African American men who have sex with other men are unaware of their seropositive status. Overall, it is estimated that fully one quarter of the 850.000-950.000 people living with HIV/AIDS in the USA are unaware that they are HIV-positive.

Sex between men remains an important aspect of the epidemic in most high-income countries. In Germany, Greece and the Netherlands, it is the most common mode of HIV transmission, while in the United State of America and in Australia it accounted for 42 per cent and 86 per cent of new HIV diagnoses, respectively. Yet. the resurgence of other sexually transmitted infections in Australia, Japan. Western Europe and the United States of America points to a revival of high-risk sexual behaviour—especially among young people, including men who have sex with men. 'The prevention programmes that had achieved notable success in limiting HIV transmission in the 1990s, especially among men who have sex with men, appear to have been shifted to the back burner in many high-income countries.

CHAPTER 2

Vulnerable India

As is elswhere, HIV/AIDS has quickly emerged as one of the most serious public health problems in India with infections currently being reported in all states and territories. India has the largest number of people living with HIV/AIDS in Asia. Globally, it is second only to South Africa in terms of the overall number of people living with the AIDS.

It is remarkable to note that the first case of AIDS in India was detected in 1986. According to UNAIDS estimates of 2001, 3.97 million Indians were HIV positive. However, due to the country's large population, the high number of infections translates into a relatively low adult prevalence of 0.8 per cent. One per cent increase in prevalence could add 5 million new infections. Health officials concede that these estimates represent only a fraction of total AIDS morbidity in India. Some experts believe the number of individuals infected with HIV/AIDS in India is actually much higher. Common opportunistic infections (OIs) associated with the reported cases of AIDS in India have been tuberculosis, fungal infection of the mouth (oral candidiasis), *Cryptosporidia* (causing diarrhoea). *Pnuemocystis carineii* (causing pneumonia) and *Herpes Zoster* (causing shingles). Managing the dual epidemic of tuberculosis and HIV/AIDS is currently posing a great challenge to the public health practitioners. HIV prevalence ranging from 10 to 20 per cent has been recorded among samples of urban TB patients in India, and it is projected that 20-25 per cent of the increase in TB cases over the next five years could be directly attributable to co-infection.

TABLE 1

HIV/AIDS Cases in India (2001)

Estimated number of adults and children living with HIV/AIDS (end 2001)	3.970.000
Total population (2001)	1.025.096.000
Adult HIV prevalence (end 2001)	0.8
HIV-1 sero-prevalence in urban areas Population most at risk (i.e., sex workers and clients, patients seeking care for a sexually transmitted infection. or others with known risk factors)	4.8%
Population not at risk (i.e., pregnant women, blood donors, or others with no known risk factors)	0.1%

Sources: UNAIDS, U.S. Census Bureau

No single state or union territory in India is free from HIV. The states and union territories can be broadly classified into three groups based on the different stages of development of the HIV epidemic.

They are:

(i) *States with generalised HIV epidemic:* In this

category are included Maharashtra, Tamil Nadu. Karnataka. Andhra Pradesh, Manipur and Nagaland where HIV prevalence has reached 1 per cent in antenatal clinic attending women representing female general population. While the first outbreak of HIV infection happened among injection heroin users in the north-eastern states of Manipur and Nagaland which have common borders with Myanmar, the other states in this category had seen the epidemic taking off first among female sex workers. However, all the states subsequently saw a significant progress of HIV in general population. HIV care and management-needs are pressing issues now in these states on top of prevention, as increasing numbers of AIDS deaths, young widows and AIDS orphans on the one hand and increased hospital bed occupancy for HIV disease on the other, are being recorded.

(ii) *Concentrated HIV epidemic states:* HIV has infected more than 5 per cent of the population group observing high-risk behaviour in these states but the prevalence in female general population has remained below 1 per cent, Gujarat, Goa, Pondicherry, Mizoram and West Bengal fall in this category. The epidemic is making in-roads in bridge population such as migrant labourers and clients of female sex workers in these states. It is still not clear what are the best ways to intervene in these populations, essentially due to lack of evidence on best practices. It is important to note that although HIV epidemic took off at the same time in IDUs in three north-eastern states (Manipur, Mizoram and Nagaland), the subsequent course taken by the virus was different, as reflected by the current sentinel surveillance data. While Manipur and Nagaland have seen a rise in HIV in IDUs followed by a rise in HIV prevalence in antenatal clinic attending women, Mizoram saw a plateauing of HIV epidemic among IDUs around 5 per cent, and HIV prevalence among heterosexuals went up. It is important to identify the determinants of this heterogeneity in different north-eastern states for effective future interventions.

(iii) *Low HIV epidemic:* Remaining states and union territories fall in this category where the population groups observing high-risk behaviour is yet to attain a 5 per cent prevalence of HIV. While these could be seen as states having windows of opportunity for preventing an intense, HIV epidemic, one needs to also examine whether the required coverage is being met under the sentinel surveillance. For example, the National AIDS Control Organisation (NACO) sees strengthening of sentinel surveillance in Assam. Bihar and Orissa as an issue of urgent importance, since in many rounds of sentinel surveillance the requisite number of samples tested (denominator) could not be collected. Although Tripura--the smallest northern state of India--which has common border with Bangladesh, has reported low HIV and limited injection drug use, anecdotal data reveals an established route for cross border smuggling of injection tidigesic (buprenorphine) ampoules from India to Bangladesh. On the other hand, Meghalaya has reported mostly oral dextropropoxyphene, diazepam and nitrazepam use and limited heroin smoking and still lower injecting practices among local youths as well as students coming from other northeastern states to Shillong for pursuing higher studies. A regional approach to designing innovative interventions is therefore required where AusAID and Sida have taken some important initiatives. However, there are states in north-east India such as Arunachal Pradesh. Tripura and Assam that are yet to get adequate attention from donor agencies for designing of intervention low prevalence setting. Similarly, diffusion of injection drug use occurring in other metropolitan cities of India outside the northeast, require urgent attention too.

Remarkably, whereas the socio-economic impact is directly linked to the magnitude of the epidemic, the extent of devastation caused by it can be gleaned from a very early study clone by Bloom and Glied. This study estimated that there will be a total of 1 million AIDS cases by the year 2000, yielding a total of $11 billion in direct and indirect costs. Direct costs include medical costs whereas indirect costs comprise value of income foregone because of AIDS-related morbidity and mortality.

No doubt, the AIDS surveillance system in India is in a nascent stage compared to the HIV surveillance system, and thus the reported cumulative AIDS cases of 20,304 greatly understates the real number of AIDS cases in India, and therefore will also understate the macro costs of the epidemic. Evidence indicates that at least 40 per cent of the patients reporting for the first time in OPDs in apex hospitals, are in advanced stages of AIDS, and are being missed out at the district levels. Thus, the figure of 1 million AIDS cases in 2000 may be much closer to the actual load of AIDS cases in the country. Murray and Lopez of the Burden Of Disease in India, the World Bank have calculated the trends in Disability Adjusted Life Years

(DALYs) lost due to selected diseases in four States (Andhra Pradesh, Karnataka, Punjab and West Bengal) of India. The study indicates that communicable diseases still predominate in terms of disease burden, especially in the young age groups. A projection till 2020 based on alternative assumptions indicate that DALYs lost due to HIV infections in India are expected to rise significantly up to the year 2010 and decline thereafter.

The impact of the epidemic is likely to be felt on all sectors households, communities, industry, agriculture, health as well as the government. A study that looked at the economic impact on individuals who were HIV positive indicated that the group on an average spent between 10 to 30 per cent of their annual incomes on HIV-related health expenditures, with the bulk of expenditures being on drugs and medicines. As expected, individuals with lower income as well as with at least one child had a greater probability of a more severe impact than other did. The immediate implication of this is that economic impact will be most severely felt by households that are relatively less well off and have a greater number of dependents. The 1997 World Bank report on Confronting AIDS states that if India maintains its current level of health care subsidies a severe AIDS epidemic would increase government expenditure by about $2 billion per year by 2010. If subsidies are increased to the 50 per cent level, the same size epidemic would increase annual government health expenditure by an additional $30 billion.

Another study which looked at the health and treatment costs for 1999 calculated that Rs. 2.045 crores would have been spent in 1999 in India, which translates into about $95 million in current prices. This was the minimum expenditures or costs that would have taken place in one year if only 2.8 per cent of the individuals are on antiretroviral treatment and only half of the new infections in 1999 display any opportunistic infection. Clearly, this kind of expenditure is untenable for a country like India, irrespective of who spends the money.

The socio-economic impact will be felt at both the individual and household level, but also at the macro and sectoral level. The two sectors that are most severely going to be affected are the health and the government sectors. The health sector will increasingly see a rise in demand for health care, and given the current health sector scenario, pressures on existing government hospitals will rise: there is already evidence of this from states like Tamil Nadu and Manipur. This is bound to have impact on individuals accessing health care for other diseases as AIDS care can crowd out not-AIDS care.

The government will also need to think strategically about its policy on newer treatments like anti-retroviral therapy (ART), which are now seen as being central to the treatment of HIV positive patients. The issue around ART has become even more critical since the prices of these drugs have been falling, indicting a possibility of subsidizing these drugs. The fact that most of the major drug companies manufacturing these drugs are Indian has made this issue even more sensitive in India.

Given India's low per capita income, as well as competing needs outside health sector--and within the health sector--it is not clear to what extent the government can subsidize ART. At the same time, greater access to ART will clearly reduce health expenditures and reduce economic impact at all levels, by keeping individuals healthy and productive. This is an area, which has yet to see much policy-oriented analysis.

While most of the public health experts and social scientists in the country believe that HIV is not going to take a course similar to the one that happened in Africa, the epidemiological evidence obtained so far does ring an alarm of concern. The virus in India has taken different courses in different states since its first detection in 1986 in Chennai and has contributed to the heterogeneous picture of the epidemic within the country. Of course, this heterogeneity has been influenced by varied sexual and injection behaviour patterns among network population groups as well as 'bridge population' linking different networks.

Genesis and extent of response to the epidemic differed across states, and played their role in shaping the epidemic differently in different states. It is important to note that the number of people living with HIV in South and South-East Asia is dominated by India; in 2001. 63 per cent of the Asia-Pacific total estimate of 6.1 million People Living with HIV (PLWH) were in this country alone. The estimated number of people living with HIV in the country was 3.5 million. 3.7 million. 3.86 million and 3.97 million respectively in 1998, 1999. 2000 and 2001.

These estimates have used HIV sentinel surveillance data collected from antenatal clinic attending women, STD clinic attendees, injecting drug users and men having sex with men. Altogether 237 select sites were used for this purpose from all over the country, of which 109 were STD clinics. 110 clinics for pregnant women, 11 sites for injecting drug users (IDUs) and only two for men having sex with men.

AIDS cases were not included at the time of calculating the estimates using sentinel surveillance data, and the age range in focus was 15 to 49 years. Also, sex workers are not currently being included as a sentinel group in the surveillance. Lack of adequate representation of all the risk groups as well as lack of proper geographic spread -- including proper representation from rural areas -- in sentinel surveillance, clearly highlight the need for involving these sub-populations and non-government organisations having active contact with some of the 'hard to reach population' such as IDUs and MSMs in surveillance activities.

HIV Transmission Modes

It is observed that in India, 75 to 80 per cent of HIV transmission is through heterosexual sex. HIV prevalence rates are highest among sex workers and their clients. The latter, in turn, take the disease back to their homes and infect their wives. Mobile populations, notably truckers, have been especially important in spreading the disease. Apart from sex workers and truckers, high-risk populations include migrant labourers, prisoners, and military troops stationed in remote areas, especially in the north-east.

Prostitution

A countrywide surveillance for HIV was initiated in 1985 by the apex research institute ICMR. This generated the first evidence for presence of HIV from a group of female sex workers in Chennai in 1986. Subsequently HIV prevalence in sex workers in Mumbai went up from 0 per cent in 1987 to 20 per cent within a period of three years. All these early cross-sectional findings prompted launching of targeted interventions in brothel based sex workers in different parts of India, especially since evidence from successful AIDS control projects around the world showed targeted intervention approach to be able to stop the transmission of infection within and from the 'core transmitters'. However, adequate knowledge of the vulnerability of certain population groups such as unorganised sector of sex workers to HIV and STD is still lacking. Thus, it is not clear how exactly to reduce risks in these hard-to-reach populations, and what would comprise effective intervention for these groups.

Drug Use

During the initial phase of HIV epidemic in India, injection drug use related HIV was identified from the north-eastern States of Manipur. Mizorum and Nagaland, which had a common international border with Myanmar; the drug of choice for injecting was heroin. The HIV prevalence in local IDUs in Manipur, Mizoram and Nagaland subsequently stabilised at 80 per cent, 5 per cent and 50 per cent respectively. Although the present scenario of drug use in the country has changed considerably, the State AIDS Prevention and Control Societies in the stares other than the North-East are yet to support outreach and harm reduction activities. Recent data from the 'Rapid Situation Assessment' reveal that a diffusion of injection drug use has taken place in major metropolitan cities of Kolkata, Delhi. Chennai and Mumbai, as well as in other parts of India over the last ten years.

The drug of choice for injecting in IDUs in these cities is Buprenorphine, and it is frequently cocktailed with sedative and anti-histaminic injections leading to venous thrombosis and abscess formation; the HIV prevalence varies from 1 per cent in IDUs of Kolkata to 31 per cent in Chennai. The reported high needle syringe sharing rate among IDUs and observed switching of large number of heroin smokers to injection drug use during heroin-drought in these cities, indicate the need for large scale intervention. Research should also be conducted to identify the factors responsible for heterogeneity in HIV prevalence among

IDUs in these cities so that appropriate intervention could be designed and national response to HIV in IDUs could be augmented.

HIV Epidemic among Children

The latest sentinel surveillance data from ante-natal clinics in seven metro citizen the country reveal that HIV infection has crossed 2 per cent in Mumbai, is more than 1 per cent in Hyderabad, Bangalore, Chennai and below 1 per cent in Kolkata, Ahmedabad and Delhi. This clearly indicates that the cities with 1 per cent or more HIV prevalence among pregnant women have already fallen under the grip of HIV epidemic in pediatric population as well. It has also been recorded that Manipur--which had the earliest explosive HIV epidemic in among IDUs--has started seeing the impact of the disease in the form of many AIDS orphans, a phenomenon which needs a very different set of interventions not yet witnessed on a large scale. The government of India has taken commendable steps in launching hospital-based prevention of HIV transmission from pregnant mothers to children through administration of short course AZT in 11 centres located in the worst hit States. However it is worth noting that two-thirds or more of the deliveries take place at husbands' or parents' homes of the pregnant women. Moreover, stigma and discrimination often come in the way of positive women accessing health care, especially in government facilities. A national feasibility study of administering short-term AZT intervention among HIV-infected mothers to prevent mother-to-child transmission of HIV was conducted between April 2000 and July 2001. The study was conducted from 11 medical institutes in five States (Maharashtra, Tamil Nadu, Andhra Pradesh. Karnataka and Manipur) in India. It was observed that a total of 192474 women were offered HIV counselling and testing services during the study period, of which 171471 (89 per cent) received the services. There was a further decline in HIV test uptake; 103,681 among 171,471 (60 per cent) undertook HIV test of which 1724 (1.7 per cent) were HIV positive. Despite best possible efforts of health care providers backed up by counselling services in the medical institutes--some of the HIV positive women in the study never came back for the test results and only 44 per cent (751/1,724) took AZT prophylaxis which was to be received from the study centres.

This further emphasises the need for innovative community-based approach for prevention of third wave of the epidemic in the pediatric population in the country. Future programme planning should look for alternate ways of reaching out to 'mothers-in-need' especially through involvement of non-government and community based organisations.

Migration

Migration has added another dimension to the epidemic in India. The country has seen--and continues to see--significant migration, both between states, and between the country and other neighbouring countries. Nepal and Bangladesh have extremely porous international borders with India. While Bangladesh still has a low HIV epidemic, the HIV prevalence among sex workers in Nepal has reached 16 per cent and among IDUs 50 per cent. Some of the destination states of India also happen to be those registering high HIV prevalence.

These include the more industrialised States of Maharashtra, Gujarat and Andhra Pradesh. These States attract male and female labourers from all over the country, but particularly from those States with lower income levels such as Uttar Pradesh, Bihar, Rajasthan and Madhya Pradesh. While these latter states have relatively low levels of reported HIV infection, labour migration to high prevalence states may soon change the scenario. Indeed many of the migrating men leave their wives and families behind thus increasing the likelihood that they will visit sex workers during their stays away from home. Migration due to various factors such as eviction of tribal people from forests to he owned by government in Rajasthan or fatal ethnic clash in Manipur have also been documented as reasons why women are forced to take up prostitution as alternate means of living.

Blood Safety

The cornerstone of programmes to reduce HIV transmission by transfusion of blood/blood product is the testing of all blood donations for HIV antibody. Although the situation has improved in India after the Supreme Court verdict in this direction, 100 per cent safe blood/ blood product transfusion is yet to be achieved in India. The main issue is of supply, demand always exceeds supply and currently only 60 per cent of the demand is being met through official sources, which has serious implications for HIV transmission in the country. States with relatively less developed rural areas and difficult hilly terrain with inadequate health care delivery services have this as a problem, but also in states such as Mumbai and West Bengal, concerns have been raised in this regard. As centralised blood transfusion services would be difficult in as vast a country as India where these are operated by government, voluntary and commercial establishments, and development of standardised processes and centralised quality assurance programmes have been recommended.

Additional inputs that could boost up the whole prevention programme in the country in this field are training of health care providers on 'rational use of blood transfusion,' 'component therapy instead of whole blood transfusion' and innovative donor deferral criteria in conjunction with blood screening. While the issues discussed above may seem diverse, needing completely separate sets of interventions, there are some fundamental commonalties underlying the spread of the virus which call out for a developmental approach to interventions. In India the major route of transmission is sexual, followed by infected blood and blood products. Taking the sexual route of transmission first, given the age structure of the population, a large majority of India's population is in the sexually active a group (49.5 per cent in the age group 15--49 as reported in NFHS-2). This figure is about 6 percentage points higher in the urban areas than in the rural areas, indicating possibly migration. Another point to rote is that all of India has an adverse sex ratio, which deteriorated further by 2001; thus there are fewer females per 1,000 males. Secondly, a slightly lower proportion of female aged 6 and above have never married compared to males.

Women in India marry at much younger ages than men, and both men and women marry at younger ages in rural than in urban areas. To really understand the extent of risky behaviour of individuals, one also needs some estimates of premarital, extra-marital as well as sexual behaviour of never-married individuals. While these figures are not easily available, it can only be conjectured that these practices exist just like anywhere else in India as well. In any case, these demographic facts do indicate the wide prevalence of marriage as well as the vulnerability of women in India, two facts that are very important in the context of the HIV/AIDS epidemic.

It also implies that it is *possible* for this sub-population of sexually active individuals to acquire the infection, though the *probability* will depend on their specific risk behaviours. While there exists now a large amount of literature on who, why and how risky sex behaviour occurs, the simple fact is that risky sex can occur only in one of two ways: deliberately (with correct knowledge) or non-deliberately. While no statistics exist on the proportion of each, it may be safe to conclude that most individuals have a long time horizon and will not wilfully engage in behaviour that may jeopardize his/her life.

However, there are some factors that may increase even this kind of behaviour, and these factors have to do with a much shorter time horizon (i.e. they do not care too much about the future) emanating from a variety of reasons, or a lifestyle that has little to offer by way of a peaceful and stable existence. But, a majority of risk behaviour is undertaken with lack of knowledge about the implication of such behaviour.

Thus we need to answer two additional questions in turn:

- Who are least likely to be informed?
- Who are most likely to have a shorter time horizon?

  It is our contention that there are a number of factors that need to be considered to address these questions, and these are the commonalties that cut across risk groups and behaviour and these are indicated below:

- *Poverty:* one of the main reasons for poverty is unemployment and/or underemployment. In addition, the poor will also include seasonally employed, a large section of the informal sector workers, beggars, street children. sex workers, slum dwellers.

- Illiterate, uneducated and less educated.
- Marginalised and disempowered populations: the poor, the uneducated, women, minorities, refugees, street children, beggars, sexual minorities.
- Those with interrupted family lives either by lifestyle choice or by force of circumstances: migrants, frequent; long-distance travellers, armed forces, refugees, slum dwellers.
- Women, especially those who are poor, uneducated, unemployed and generally disempowered due to the cultural and patriarchal structures of Indian society.
- The youth and the elderly, especially those belonging to any of the vulnerable groups mentioned above Many of these factors go into making a large majority of India's population *potentially* vulnerable to HIV via the sexual route of transmission.

Care and Support

A few organisations such as the HIV/AIDS Alliance and Naz India are filling this gap in three states of Andhra Pradesh, Tamil Nadu and Delhi through their network of implementing partner organisations. The needs include medical support, counselling, livelihood, educational support and working with the families and communities to reduce stigma and discrimination. It is being increasingly realised that care can be given at home and not necessarily in an institutional setting.

It is now necessary to focus attention on innovative ways of extending support to those affected, without injecting elements of inequity across socioeconomic classes or across disease categories. Replicable and feasible models of care and support need to be developed. One important lacuna so far in the care and support efforts have been a lack of legal framework, which ensures the rights of PLWHA, especially in the areas of workplace and health care settings.

Responses

India's AIDS programmes are implemented through the National AIDS Control Organisation (NACO), a semi-independent organisation established in 1992 within the Health Ministry. Its special status was intended to prevent the bureaucratic delays that normally plague India's decision-making process.

India's National AIDS Control Policy adheres to the following strategy in its effort to prevent and control HIV/AIDS throughout the country:

(i) Prevent the further spread of the disease by:
   (a) Controlling sexually transmitted infections and promoting condom use: and
   (b) Improving HIV/AIDS awareness and providing people with the necessary tools to protect themselves:
   (c) Ensuring the availability of safe blood and blood products.

(ii) Create a socioeconomic environment that enables individuals to protect themselves from infection and allows families and communities to provide care and support to people living with HIV/AIDS.

(iii) Improve services--both in hospitals and through community-based home care--that provide care for people living with HIV/AIDS.

The National AIDS Control Organisation, with financial assistance from the World Bank, is currently implementing the second phase of its National AIDS Control Programme. The objectives of this phase are to:

- Reduce the spread of HIV infection in at-risk populations;
- Reduce the spread of HIV in the general population;
- Strengthen the impact and sustainability of national. state, and local HIV/AIDS programmes;
- Build capacity to provide low-cost, community-based care; and
- Promote intersectoral links to combat HIV/AIDS.

NACO put froward a the National AIDS Control Programme (NACP)--a fully centrally-sponsored scheme--which comprises Surveillance, Programme Management, Information, Education and Communication (IEC), Blood Safety, Condom Promotion, Control of STDs, and Clinical Management. Needless to say, much less was known about the determinants and outcome of HIV/AIDS at that point than is known now.

This first phase (1992-1999) of the project was mainly to be financed by a Government of India contribution of $14.1 million, an IDA credit of $84 million and a WHO co-financing grant of $1.5 million. It should be noted that the GOI contribution was actually much higher than the original estimate and came to $27.5 million. In addition, there were two important additional sources of financing: USAID and DFID. Now, in Phase 2 of the NACP. the objectives of NACO continue to be similar; these are:

- To reduce spread of HIV infection.
- To strengthen India's capacity to respond to HIV/AIDS on a long-term basis.

The targets envisaged in the NACP-2 are the following:

- Reduce blood-borne transmission of HIV to less than 1 per cent of total transmissions.
- To introduce Hepatitis C as the fifth mandatory test for blood screening.
- To set up new and upgrade existing blood banks as well blood component separation units.
- To attain awareness level of at least 90 per cent among youth and those in reproductive ages.
- Training of NGOs for targeted intervention programmes among high risk groups, to in turn promote condom use to at least 90 per cent in these groups.
- Conduct annual Family Health Awareness Campaigns among general population: provision of drugs for control of STDs and RTIs.
- Promotion of voluntary testing facilities so that every district in the country will have at least one voluntary testing facility.
- Use of interactive awareness campaigns like folk arts and street theatre.
- Cover all the schools and universities under awareness programmes.
- Promote organisations of PLWHA and give then financial support to form self-help groups. The above are firm targets that the NACP-II hopes to achieve by the end of 2004. Further, the major components of NACP-II under which these targets would be achieved are:

  (i) *Priority targeted interventions for high risk population:* this has to be done mainly through NGOs/CBOs/Public sector.

(ii) *Preventive interventions for the general population:* this has to be done through IEC, awareness campaigns, voluntary testing and counselling (VTC), reduction or transmission by infected blood and blond products and prevention of occupational exposure.

(iii) *Low cost care for people living with HIV/AIDS:* financial and technical assistance to be provided to states/UTs for home-based and community-based care.

(iv) Institutional strengthening including strengthening surveillance activities and research and development.

(v) *Inter-sectoral collaboration:* coordination within the Ministry of Health and Family Welfare, as well as other central ministries.

The main emphasis on NACP-II is on clean and adequate supply of blood, IEC and targeted interventions among high risk groups. The achievements of the first phase however lie in responding swiftly, building programme capacity, efforts to tone up the surveillance system, getting the blood banks to supply cleaner blood and raising awareness. A major innovation in Phase I of NACP was the replacement of the earlier structure of State AIDS Cell by State AIDS Control Society. This step was taken to ensure easier disbursement of funds, lack of delays and more decentralisation in decisionmaking. The other has been to move from developing and disseminating IEC materials to actually translating these into action by using the targeted intervention approach.

Prevention among low-risk groups is to receive the highest allocation (33.7 per cent), followed by institutional strengthening and prevention among high-risk groups (24.8 per cent and 23 per cent respectively). Out of the total Rs. 1155.1 crores in the NACP- II. World Bank has provided Rs. 959.1 crores; the remaining Rs. 196 crores is to be provided by the Government of India. In other words, the World Bank is to provide 83 per cent of the proposed outlay for NACP-II. In addition to these two sources of funding, the two other major sources of funding are USAID and DFID. The USAID has extended support of Rs. 166 crores, to the Government of Maharashtra for implementation of AVERT project, based on the earlier success of the still on-going APAC project in Tamil Nadu. DFID has given assistance of Rs. 104 crores, for Sexual Health projects in the states of Andhra Pradesh, Gujarat, Kerala and Orissa.

The overall focus of the NACP is towards prevention and control: about 60 per cent of its funds are allocated to prevent the transmission of HIV. Also, the other major partners --DFID and USAID--are also heavily involved in prevention. Care and support receive a much smaller allocation--14 per cent--in the programme. In fact, the number of Targeted Interventions (TI) projects in India are 475, with the highest numbers being carried out in Tamil Nadu, followed by Maharashtra. DFID and USAID as mentioned above fund many of these.

It is interesting to note that there are no NACP-funded TI projects in the following states and UTs: Andaman & Nicobar Islands, Bihar, Dadra and Nagar Haveli. Daman and Diu. Delhi, Jammu and Kashmir, Lakshwadeep. Meghalaya, Pondicherry, Sikkim and Uttar Pradesh. However, it is also true that there are instances of non-governmental organisations running targeted interventions in different states: for example, there is an EU-funded 5-

city oral sublingual buprenorphine substitution programme for IDUs, which includes Delhi.

International Assistance

Organisations involved in both prevention and control programmes as well as care and support can be divided into four categories: the UN agencies, bilaterals, international NGOs (INGOs) and domestic NGOs/CBOs.

USAID is one of the largest donors to HIV/AIDS prevention and control programmes in the country, allocating $12.2 in 2002, an increase from $9 million in 2001. USAID/India's primary objective is to focus on HIV prevention and containment of the epidemic. Prevention activities target at risk populations, such as commercial sex workers and truck drivers, who are likely-core transmitters of HIV in India. However. USAID/India is also working to build awareness in low-risk rural-populations and will endeavour to promote prevention activities through health services outreach projects. USAID bilateral assistance is focused in Tamil Nadu and Maharashtra, states with adult prevalence greater than 1 per cent. USAID has developed a partnership approach with the Government of India, non-governmental organisations, businesses, and others to fight HIV.

Emphasis is placed on community-based and work-based approaches to controlling the epidemic. USAID began to tackle India's HIV/AIDS epidemic in 1992 with the development of the AIDS Prevention and Control (APAC) project in the southern Indian state of Tamil Nadu, one of India's recognised epicentres.

USAID expanded its programme in 1999 to include the state of Maharashtra, where antenatal HIV prevalence is approaching 2 per cent. The seven-year. $41.5 million

AVERT activity funds comprehensive prevention and care programmes throughout the state of Maharashtra. The major activities under both projects include financial and technical assistance to non-governmental organisations to undertake targeted interventions on HIV/AIDS, capacity building of health care providers, and behaviour change communication, including mass media, condom promotion, sexually transmitted infection prevention, and advocacy.

USAID increased the number of grants in 2002 to nongovernmental organisations, and began addressing new issues such as care and support for HIV-infected persons, voluntary counselling and testing, interventions with industrial workers, and geographic expansion of the APAC project to include Pondicherry, an adjacent and culturally similar area to the present activity area in Tamil Nadu.

The other USAID-funded HIV/AIDS activities include supporting the National Ports project, Project Lighthouse Implemented by Population Services International in the 12 major ports of India, this project addresses vulnerable populations associated with ports, which include casual workers, migrants, formal port employees, truckers, and commercial sex workers. The project strategies include behaviour change communication, condom promotion, and sexually transmitted infection treatment. USAID also supports Family Health International through the IMPACT project. Family Health International supports nongovernmental organisations to provide support to children infected and affected by, HIV/AIDS and other vulnerable children, pilot activities on care and support, applied research and developing models for HIV/AIDS programming.

The following include additional USAID-supported activities:

(a) *Prevention:* The 10-year. $10 million AIDS Prevention and Control project in Tamil Nadu supports non-governmental organisation efforts to design and implement community-based prevention programmes that target at-risk populations, such as sex workers and their clients, patients with sexually transmitted infections slum dwellers, and truckers and their helpers. The project emphasises preventive behaviour through peer education, the promotion of condoms, and improved treatment of sexually transmitted infections.

(b) *Capacity building:* The Mission supports the National AIDS Control Organisation by providing financial and technical assistance to national programmes. USAID also provides grants to medical colleges and institutions to improve HIV/AIDS and sexually transmitted infection training for health care providers. The AVERT project in Maharashtra state supports prevention efforts in urban and peri-urban areas and works to increase the role of non-governmental organisations in HIV prevention.

(c) *Care and support:* Through both the bilateral and field support programmes, USAID is exploring innovative models for care and support, including home and community-based care.

(d) *Protection of children affected by AIDS:* USAID supports comprehensive projects addressing the special needs of children both infected and affected by HIV/AIDS throughout the country.

(e) *Research and surveillance:* USAID funds annual HIV risk-behavioural surveillance surveys that track key behaviour changes, such as condom use, treatment-seeking of sexually transmitted infections and decreases in sexual contacts with non-regular partners. In Tamil Nadu, behavioural surveillance surveys and available seroprevalence data suggest a promising trend in that state: an increase in HIV prevention behaviour and a decrease in HIV prevalence levels. Additional clinical research activities are being planned through India CLEN.

(f) *Condoms:* To expand and improve condom distribution, USAID-supported projects provide financial support and technical assistance to the commercial sector. The programme assists the Drug Controller of India in strengthening quality control and monitoring activities, and is working with manufacturers to improve condom packaging. The programme also supports the private and commercial sectors in creating new diagnostic products and improving the quality and marketing of existing products.

International NGOs

The major bilateral players are USAID, DFID, CIDA, Sida and AusAID. European Union (EU) has also emerged as an important player. Besides these, there are other international Foundations and NGOs (INGOs) like the Ford Foundation, MacArthur Foundation, Population Council, Family Health International (FHI), HIV/AIDS Alliance etc. that have added significance to the overall activities around HIV/AIDS in India. Most of the donor interventions are in the areas of prevention through targeted interventions and awareness campaigns, and primarily focused in the states of Maharashtra, Andhra Pradesh, Tamil Nadu, Manipur, West Bengal, Kerala and Gujarat. One of the few international agencies working on HIV/AIDS care and support in India is Oxfam in Manipur and

India HIV/AIDS Alliance in the states of Andhra Pradesh, Tamil Nadu and Delhi. The states with limited donor HIV/AIDS interventions are Bihar, Rajasthan, Karnataka, Orissa, Assam, Arunachal Pradesh and Tripura. Many of these states are also underdeveloped with high levels of poverty, as discussed in the first section. Some of the other international organisations that are working on HIV/AIDS in India are CARE India who are in the process of negotiating a US $ 15-20 million grant (from USAID) to work in seven low prevalent states across the country. Their focus will be on prevention and awareness building amongst vulnerable groups. BBC World Service Trust is working on communication for the northern states of Uttar Pradesh, Rajasthan and Delhi. Catholic Relief Services, Plan International, Action AID. World Vision are other international organisations also working on HIV/AIDS who are beginning to support more prevention as well as care and support programmes in the high prevalent states.

CEDPA will be working on HIV/AIDS and youth as a part of the USAID funded IFPS project in Uttar Pradesh. Some of the other Foundations funding in India are Bill and Melinda Gates Foundation (for whom India and HIV/AIDS are becoming a key focus area), Packard Foundation (focus on Bihar and Jharkhand for reproductive health and sexuality), Francois Xavier Bagnoud (FXB), Elton John Foundation, Richard Gere Foundation, etc.

NGOs at National Level

In addition to these organisations mentioned above. India has seen an emergence of several competent NGOs who have often filled in the gaps left by other players, especially in working with vulnerable groups. While it is difficult to list all the NGOs working in India on HIV/AIDS and related issues, some of the more notable ones are Y.R.G. Care (Chennai), Indian Network of Positive People (INP+), Naz Foundation India Trust (Delhi), Sahara (Delhi), Sharan (Delhi), SPARSHA (Society for Positive Atmosphere and Related Support to HIV/AIDS, Kolkata). Freedom Foundation (Bangalore, Hyderabad), SOS Medical Foundation (Nasik), Prayas (Pune), Sangram (Sangli), CASA (Mumbai), Prepare (Chennai), Lawyers Collective (Mumbai and Delhi), Durbar Mahila Samanvaya Committee (DMSC, Kolkata) etc. In addition to these, India has seen the emergence of several NGO conglomerations such as FINGODAP, working on drug and AIDS, and India Network of NGOs (INN). The rich NGO experience unfortunately has not been adequately analysed, evaluated and documented, including showcasing of best practices.

This has meant that this resource has been both nonscalable as well as underutilised. This remains an important area where donors can step in to facilitate a wider dissemination and utilisation of knowledge, experience and best practices emanating from the NGO/CBO sector. Also, the NGOs often lack technical as well as administrative capacities, and have very little knowledge or understanding of research. The donors can help by lending technical support as we'll as research support to these organisations.

The India HIV/AIDS Alliance has been primarily focusing on care and support programmes in the states of Andhra Pradesh, Tamil Nadu and Delhi. The purpose has been to provide people living with HIV/AIDS (PLHA), children affected by AIDS (CAA) and their families with appropriate and adequate support in their clinical and psychosocial needs through the delivery of integrated home and community care by NGOs/CBOs; and to strengthen communities in their response to the epidemic and the mitigation of its impact.

The major lessons learned from the implementation experience have been that integrated community development organisations are more flexible and innovative in identifying and planning community based care and support activities, and also address stigma and discrimination, in comparison to those that have existing institutional services or are involved in prevention through targeted interventions. These organisations also address sustainability issues early on in project development. Participatory Community Assessment (PCA) and use of participatory tools is also a good start up activity for implementation of HIV/AIDS care and support projects.

APAC/VHS/USAID

AIDS Prevention and Control (APAC) project is administered by Voluntary Health Services (VHS). Chennai, with financial assistance from USAID, under a bilateral agreement with the Government of India. APAC initiated HIV/AIDS prevention in Tamil Nadu in the year 1996 with the overall goal of reducing the sexual transmission of HIV in the state. The project supports NGO partners to implement thematic intervention projects reaching "Truckers and Helpers". "Women in Prostitution", "People Living in Slums" and tourists. It also conducts HIV Behaviour Surveillance Survey (BSS) to capture the intervention efforts, and to inform the intervention programme. Altogether five rounds of BSS have been completed by now.

APAC is the only project in India that has attempted to systematically look into the changes in risk behaviour of different population groups since 1996 through 2000, and has used the behaviour surveillance data for informing interventions. The experience of APAC for tripartite collaboration and documented behaviour change are certainly worth emulating after adapting to different local conditions.

Project Concern International (PCI)

Project Concern International (PCI) has been working on HIV/ AIDS in India for the last few years. The major focus of their HIV/AIDS interventions has been behaviour change through counselling and education, condom promotion. STI treatment and counselling (syndromic management of STIs). training on STIs. HIV/AIDS and sex and sexuality. The special groups for focus are truckers, street and working children. PLHA and their families, sex workers, injecting drug users, adolescents and *devadasis*. Their HIV/AIDS care and support interventions have included home based care and support for PLHA through medical and psychosocial care, training and orientation of PLHA, their families and community members. PCI has provided a forum for NGOs to come together for discussions and experience sharing that has been beneficial for cross fertilisation of ideas and innovative intervention development. Implementation of Management Information Systems (MIS) for the partner NGOs as also financial systems that are capable of capturing information on local donation, cost recovery mechanisms, income-generating projects and community contributions have greatly enhanced the effective functioning of these NGOs.

Department for International Development (DFID)

DFID has been implementing the Sexual Health Project in West Bengal with the focus of HIV/AIDS control programmes and developing IEC techniques. DFID has also supported a national Healthy Highways Project with the truckers' community. The pilot project has been integrated into the NACPII. In addition. DFID has formulated "partnership for sexual health" projects for the prevention and control of HIV/ AIDS and other sexually transmitted infections in the states of Andhra Pradesh, Gujarat. Kerala and Orissa. The objectives of the project are:

(i) To ensure better sexual health for people vulnerable to sexually transmitted diseases (STDs) and HIV, especially the poor: and

(ii) lowering incidence of sexually transmitted infections in the four states. The components of the project are:

(a) surveillance,

(b) condom programming by ensuring that quality condoms are made available and acceptable to those who are vulnerable to STDs/HIV through effective social marketing,

(c) strengthening service providers to respond to clients needs through targeted interventions for vulnerable groups, such as sex workers and their clients, men having sex with men, migrant workers and prison inmates.

Some of the lessons learned are: political will is the essence of success of HIV/AIDS prevention programs: establishing and maintaining decision making systems needs full co-operation from the government; planning for HIV/AIDS prevention programmes at the state level needs greater co-ordination between GO-NGO: having a Management Agency makes coordination feasible; collating the strengths of each organisation is the key to success: build capacities of the states to sustain the programme which includes developing local expertise in HIV/AIDS prevention.

Role of Private Sector

In addition to the government and national and international donors and NGOs, the private sector in India has also made its presence felt in HIV prevention activities, especially around issues like workplace interventions, community programmes and support to NGOs. The Confederation of Indian Industry (CII) has supported over 1700 companies in establishing workplace programmes and has provided income generation opportunities for people living with HIV/AIDS.

B. Muthuraman, the managing director of Tata Steel, in his statement on the HIV(+) and AIDS Policy on 1 October. 2001 mentioned that Tata Steel would take measures to prevent the incidence and spread of HIV and AIDS in the society. In case of need, the company would arrange to provide counselling and medical guidance to these patients and their families. AIDS awareness and treatment of drug dependence are two other related issues that TATA has been concerned for quite some time now. Since mid-1990s Tata Steel has been providing infrastructure support for running drug detoxification centre in Barandi, Bihar where its collaborating partner organisation. The Calcutta Samaritans' is in-charge of the technical inputs as well as service provision. The changing scenario of drug use from heroin smoking to synthetic pharmaceutical injecting among the local youths including a few industrial workers in and around Jamshedpur called for such an action and the present status of this collaboration exemplifies a successful networking between private corporate sector and NGO, many of which kind should take place within the country in order to achieve a significant public health impact on HIV/AIDS prevention and care. Other examples of such activities include Tata Tea's collaboration with tea plantation workers in Kerala. Similar collaboration and business coalitions against HIV/AIDS are being set up in different states, and CII has also set up the Indian Business Trust for HIV/AIDS. In another example of donors collaborating with the private sector, the ILO in consultation with its Indian tripartite constituents and NACO has developed a three-phased programme, aimed at establishing a sustainable national action on HIV/AIDS prevention, care and support in the world of work.

The notable features of the ILO project include: guidance to the project by a high-level project management team, mobilisation of partners through stakeholders meetings and consultations/seminars, etc., in an attempt to put HIV/AIDS on the agenda, research based advocacy, documentation of corporate responses to HIV/AIDS, compilation and dissemination of existing research studies on HIV/AIDS in the world of work, initiation of action research projects and capacity building.

From the point of view of the national response, the mail strengths of NACP in India have been the following:

- swiftness of response
- setting up a fairly strong organisation like the NACO
- ability to procure in two stages a high level of funding commitment from a major organisation like the World Bank
- ability to build up state level capacities
- ability to attract additional donors and their funding
- successful collaboration with major bilaterals and INGOs
- ability to work with Indian NGOs

However, gaps remain even today in the NACP as well as in the non-government response. Most of these-gap have been recognised, but there has been an inability to deal effectively with these, mainly because of an imperfect understanding of how to move forward. Below we list some of the continued problems despite over a decade-long response:

- Inability to integrate HIV/AIDS into the mainstream of public health activities
- Inability to reduce stigma and discrimination
- Inadequate focus on vulnerability factors, especially poverty, illiteracy and disempowerment
- Inadequate geographic and population coverage in term of targeted interventions
- Inadequate focus on care and support
- Inadequate attention paid to the issues around antiretroviral treatment
- Almost complete neglect of monitoring and evaluation of programmes
- Lack of focus on generating evidence, especially around risk practices and treatment-seeking behaviour among bridge population and core transmitters.

Of these, the most damaging have been the first and the last one. It is our contention that by making HIV/AIDS a stand-alone and vertical programme, which is not integrated into an overall public health framework, we may have added to the stigma and discrimination surrounding it. The high-profile activities and funding have also brought out in sharp focus the possible inequities that such programmes might inject into both national health policy as well as overall welfare policies.

This is because, it is not always clear why HIV/AIDS should merit greater attention than other infectious diseases, or why those who are infected should merit greater assistance than those who are not infected but fatally sick. This inadequate recognition given to equity issues has been instrumental in bringing criticism to the extent that some have questioned the very need for such a high-funded project for AIDS. In addition to not adequately recognising the need for integration into other health programmes right at the outset, or even midway into the first phase, the problem was compounded by messages of IEC that made HIV and AIDS stand out like some frightening and severe malady, which happens only to those who ask for it by behaving in manners not consistent with Indian morals. To a great extent, this high profiling of the epidemic was also due to the multiplicity of players, especially the international donor communities, which poured funding into prevention and control activities. A related and equally important point is that while much of the NACO core funds as well as co-financing went into prevention and control, almost no mechanism was put in place to evaluate these prevention activities.

A prime example is IEC, which has often been implemented through targeted interventions aimed at high-risk population. There is no allocation made in the NACP budget for monitoring and evaluation. While additional funding is always welcome in a cash-strapped country, funding does not seem to be the problem in India. It is an imperfect and inadequate understanding of what works, which can come only if evaluation procedures are put in place before activities are being planned. Evaluation is a scientific process and cannot generally be done well in an ex-post fashion. Another example is the proposed scaling up of the MTCT programme, which has been put in place before any evaluation of the current programme, has been done. Unfortunately, the other donors have also not insisted in scientific evaluations, though it is being recognised now that there is a need to know whether good money is being thrown after bad programmes. As for care and support, it is clear that no single organisation or even the government can shoulder the care responsibilities of AIDS patients; it is neither feasible nor is it equitable in terms of other diseases. However, it is possible to remove the constraints in care-seeking and patient-management with careful planning, and helping groups to help themselves in planning for the future. This would, of course, require a completely new and truly developmental approach to the epidemic, requiring integration of poverty reduction and other welfare programmes into HIV/ AIDS activities.

This is again not something that has been attempted in any serious fashion. As for the national NGOs, while there are many that are doing commendable work, there is a lot going on that is not being evaluated either. If national and large donor-driven programmes are not evaluated, this is even truer of NGO activities in India. There is no monitoring and evaluation at all, especially outcome evaluation. While figures are not easily available, it is probably true that much of the funding continues to flow into behaviour change and IEC activities--an area where it is easy to put in money, but which is difficult to evaluate in terms of outcome. On the other hand, national NGOs, including some international ones with branches in India are also filling in one important gap in response--care. There are now a few NGOs and INGOs like YRG Care, Naz Foundation--India Trust, HIV AIDS Alliance, ARCON, etc., that are catering to the needs of at least a small proportion of PLWHAs. Finally, in all the programmes --national or international --there has been a lack of research component, operational or otherwise. Except for some organisations like Voluntary Health Services (VHS).

NGOs and INGOs have almost never undertaken serious research into areas of their interventions. One aspect of this omission has meant that there has been an imperfect understanding of the impact of the epidemic on different, sectors. The one that should concern India immediately is the health sector.

While the prevalence of HIV in India may seem relatively low--0.7 per cent of the general adult population compared with rates of over 20 per cent in South Africa. Zimbabwe and Botswana--the infection has now been detected in all the states and union territories. It is no longer confined to vulnerable groups such as sex workers and transport workers, or to urban areas, and here lies the necessity for urgent scaled up responses for prevention of further spread of HIV. Pilot HIV intervention projects supported by different donor agencies during phase-I of the National AIDS Control Programme (NACP) in India have identified a number of essential elements of intervention, which were incorporated in the second phase of programme planning.

However, it is important to understand that while there are some essential elements (involvement of communities, creation of enabling environment, peer-based behaviour change intervention etc) that go into any intervention, each context and setting is different, and therefore scaling up should be done with great caution. In other words, exactly the same "best practice" — for example Sonagachi sex worker intervention--when put in another setting with all the essential elements in place may not yield the same outcomes.

There may be a number of reasons why scaling-up and

replication has not happened — even for some of the best practices. While a few such practices have been documented, inadequate attention has been paid to producing a complete blue print of these interventions.

There are several interventions carried out by a multiplicity of agencies and organisations all ever India. However, there has been very little documentation of these interventions. Without mapping the universal set of interventions, it is not possible to take the next step of evaluating which of these actually work.

Inadequate current response to HIV/AIDS in India stems from the fact that the knowledge base about the epidemic is far from perfect. There are some critical gaps in information with regard to:

- HIV/STD Surveillance in female sex workers, low risk male population groups and migrant labourers
- Countrywide mapping of HIV/AIDS interventions in prevention as well as care and support
- Treatment seeking behaviour of vulnerable groups such as sex workers and IDUs
- Risk practices and treatment seeking behaviour of bridge population
- Socio-economic impact on households, various sectors especially the health sector and the economy as a whole
- Cost-effectiveness of interventions.

For informed and effective policymaking, it is imperative to start generating evidence in these areas. The information can be generated by a wide variety of organisations and by using various methods, including operations research. It must be pointed out here that good research on the epidemic must always be based on the involvement of HIV-affected individuals.

India has been able to respond fairly quickly and comprehensively to the AIDS epidemic. However, there are still many areas where more focus and attention are required. The main lacunae in the current collective response has been that despite a recognition of the need to mainstream, strategies of poverty reduction and prevention and control and care and support have remained more or less parallel. Thus, the Planning Commission has yet to take a serious note of the epidemic and the need for integrating responses with other developmental ones. This lack of mainstreaming has also resulted in a paradoxical situation, where too much visibility accorded to HIV/AIDS has added to the stigma and discrimination by creating a mysterious world around the epidemic. This could be eliminated or at least reduced only by an approach which recognises that for successful prevention and control it is essential to pay attention to vulnerability factors, especially poverty, illiteracy and disempowerment.

The other shortfall of the current response is the geographic gaps that exist in prevention and control measures: while some states and areas have received a lot of focus, others have received very little. Thus, for instance, some of the most underdeveloped states like Orissa and Bihar have very little happening there compared to states like Tamil Nadu and Maharashtra. The low prevalence in these states is absolutely misleading because of the many vulnerability factors that make them potentially susceptible to high rates of transmission. Another feature of the current response is the almost complete omission of monitoring and evaluation of programmes; there are very few interventions that have been accompanied by-evaluation to see whether these work and to what extent. This is potentially a worrying situation since resources are scarce, and there *is* the danger that more resources will be spent on programmes that do not work very well.

In general there has been a lack of focus on generating evidence, especially around risk practices and treatment-seeking behaviour among bridge population and core transmitters. There is therefore the need to compile best practices in different types of interventions, from the point of view of scalability. Based on these conclusions, we present the recommendations and priorities below.

General Priorities

(i) *Emphasis on both prevention and control as well as care and support: the* epidemic has been around for more than 15 years now in India. But infections continue to occur in new areas and new groups, clearly indicating the need for continued efforts on prevention. At the same time, the need for care and support of those affected has increased enormously. Therefore donors should still treat prevention as their primary focus. At the same time, it should increasingly try to find innovative ways of dealing with issues of care and support.

(ii) *Scaling up:* the following are essential components that need focus before scaling up.

- mapping of interventions across the country
- analysis and documentation of what works
- estimation of size of vulnerable groups, especially overlooked groups like unorganised sex workers in cabin-restaurants
- constraints faced in increasing coverage through scaled up responses

(iii) *Priorities under prevention:* these are some of the key issues that need to be considered.

- *Low risk population:* situational analysis, operational research and interventions for the following groups -- clients of sex workers, spouse of IDUs, migrant labourers and slum population.
- *Bridge population:* determinants of risk-taking behaviour and treatment seeking behaviour of bridge populations like truck drivers. Innovative ways of reaching out to these groups.
- *Informal and unorganised sector workers:* collaboration and cooperation with the private corporate sector to bring these hard-to-reach workers under the umbrella of prevention.
- *Third wave of HIV among pediatric population:* design appropriate interventions based on evidence from feasibility study that indicates reasons why most of the mothers do not access institution based interventions.
- *Cross border,* cross country collaboration to address vulnerability issues of migrant population and girls engaged in prostitution, between India and neighbouring countries like Nepal and Bangladesh.
- *Adolescents and youth:* situation analysis, operational research and appropriate interventions for this group.
- *Capacity building for effective transfusion services:* innovative blood donor deferral and training of health care providers for rational use of blood transfusion as well as component therapy, as opposed to whole blood transfusion.

(iv) *Priorities under care and support:* very little is known about how best to carry out care and support programmes. Thus, the following are identified areas:

- research on socioeconomic impact, especially for households and communities, including quality and accessibility of antiretroviral therapy, and exploring mechanisms like health insurance to support increased health expenditure.
- how to foster involvement of people living with HIV/ AIDS and their friends.
- Models for best practices in care and support, including costing.

(v) *Research needs:* there is a need to document good research as well as support research for generating knowledge. Such research can be used by funding agencies including NACO to inform policy.

Some of the areas of research are:

- Links between poverty and other developmental factors on the one hand and HIV/AIDS on the other: this will enable answering questions like who needs what type of help, and how. The priority areas mentioned under prevention are also areas of research that can be focused upon.

(vi) Impact of morbidity and mortality on the health sector: Implications for the dual epidemic of HIV and TB in India: monitoring of trend of resistance in isolates of *mycobacterium tuberculosis.*

(vii) *Geographic focus:* focus on areas/states that have received little attention so far from government and other donors/ NGOs.

- Need to extend analysis and coverage of areas that see out-migration to high-prevalence states in India, for example Bihar and Orissa are prime examples of neglected but vulnerable states.
- Diffusion of injection drug use in metropolitan cities of India and heterogeneity in HIV prevalence in IDUs.

(viii) Monitoring and evaluation (M & E)

- Strengthen capacity for M & E of programmes and projects
- Advocacy for M & E activities
- Training in-house as well as outside on M & E.
- Lend technical support on M & E to NACO as well as other donors.

(ix) *Capacity building;* stress should be placed on involving communities infected and affected by HIV/AIDS.

- Roadmap for peer outreach intervention
- Training to build capacity for operational research
- Enhancing research and analysis capacities of NGOs as well as private corporate sector
- Training, orientation and sensitisation of personnel of concerned ministries and departments, such as health, home, education, labour, industry etc. This will also enhance inter-sectoral collaboration.

II

HIV/AIDS and Children: Conspiracy of Silence

Children with perinatally acquired HIV tend to survive upto their middle childhood or adolescence stage, though this case, is seen in many of them but not all (Black, 1990). Consequently, the disclosure of HIV/AIDS to a child who has diagnosed positive is becoming an increasingly common clinical issue. As some family members have been reluctant to discuss the nature of the illness with their infected child or adolescent, this encourages to look into the matter of disclosure of illness to HIV-infected children and adolescents (Black, 1990). Considerable guidelines exist about the disclosure of a chronic illness to a child. In general, disclosure is geared to a child's level of cognitive development and psychosocial maturity. For most illnesses, young children receive simple explanations about the nature of their illness and what their responsibilities are in caring for themselves.

A couple says,

> *"we ignored safe sex often and we are leaving orphans behind ..."*

Mother aged 38 years, HIV positive,

> " . . . I *am keeping my 6 years old child in child-care center and I do not have any future plan for my child . . ."*

Another mother aged 40 years, HIV positive,

> *" ... I do not have any property to keep my child under any guardian, probably I will keep my child with her grandmother aged 65 years ..."*

In general, the above cases reflect that PLHAs' failure to develop a permanency plan (create a will identifying a legal guardian for their children) further complicates this issue, particularly for children who are HIV infected. Development of a permanency plan and providing continuum of care are challenging tasks for parents with HIV/AIDS for numerous reasons. These reasons includes denial of the severity of illness, fear of disclosure, health status of parent and HIV infected child, lack of reliable adult to provide care, psychological adjustment of parents and domestic violence in the home. Loss of parents and changes in caregivers interfere with mastery of developmental milestones and coping abilities of children and adolescents.

One of the HIV positive women, 22 years old, stated, -

> *"my child is seven years old. She is too small to understand the details of the disease. Just as we explain in simple terms when children get fever, cold etc. I have told her ..."*

Another woman who has a 13-year-old son says,

> *"My son is growing up and I think he is quite matured and understanding one of these days. I am planning to explaining him about everything patiently ...* so *that he can take care of his two younger sisters.. ."*

A man who is HIV positive, aged 37 years, said,

> *"my daughter is 12 years and she has now began asking me several questions about the illness. But I feel I am not so well informed. So I am planning to take her to "didi' (Counsellor of NGO) and ask her to explain ..."*

On the other hand, two street children (aged 15 and 16 years) said that they were aware of the illness, the causes, the course and the impact of the disease.

> *"We do not bother about this HIV and all. We just take 'ganja' or drink and enjoy the life ..."*

The discussion of exact diagnosis and prognosis of the disease are not very important at an early age with young children of 6-15 years. But, as the children mature, they should be fully informed of the nature and consequences of their illness and should be encouraged to actively participate in their own medical care. Many studies proved that children have exhibited better coping skills and fewer psychosocial problems when appropriately informed about the nature and consequences of their illness (Haroon and Viloari, 2002).

Nevertheless, some parents and health care professionals are reluctant to inform children about their HIV/AIDS status. Some of the reasons given by family members for not disclosing HIV/AIDS status are concerns about the impact of disclosure on a child's emotional health and fear by the parents that knowledge will negatively affect a child's 'will' to live. Additional reasons often given by parents of HIV-infected children include, a sense of guilt about having transmitted infection to the child, anger of the child when learning about his/her perinatal transmission, difficulty in coping with their own infection with HIV/ AIDS and fear of inadvertent disclosure by the child. Disclosure of status by the children may lead to stigmatization, discrimination, or ostracism toward the children and other family members. This reflects that families are also concerned about the difficulty of children in keeping a secret and therefore limiting the disclosure to only selected persons.

Denial is common, and parents may not be able to deal with their own HIV status or that of a family member. Accepting the full consequences of HIV/AIDS within the family and learning to cope can be a lengthy process for (any) individuals. Failure to cope with HIV/AIDS appropriately may signify psychosocial dysfunction that needs specific counselling and therapy for parents. Though parents may be making requests for non-disclosure based on what they believe is best for their children, physicians also have a responsibility to make an independent assessment of a child's readiness for disclosure.

One of the couples, HIV positive, expressed,

> *"... we feel so guilty of having passed on the infection to our child. So we have no courage or the heart to sit face to face with him and tell about the problem. Let time and life take its own course and I am sure someday somehow he'll understand ..."*

Another mother aged 33, HIV positive, stated,

> *"she is old (aged 13 years) enough to understand. But, I do not know how she will react. I am scared she may feel sad and depressed or probably may get so angry and take an extreme step such as running away or committing suicide. Then what we do. So I am not telling her ..."*

One of the mothers aged *29,* HIV positive, stated,

> *"I want to tell her. But she is so friendly and sociable with everyone that I fear she may withdraw from interacting with others ..."*

The concern of families that lies behind concealing information is protecting their children from certain problems but in the process, they often tend to fall at risk of encountering other unforeseen problems. Children may develop inappropriate and hurtful fantasies about their illness. A 'conspiracy of silence' surrounding children infected with HIV/AIDS may isolate them from potential sources of social support. In the unfortunate event of the death of a parent, the opportunity is lost for children to discuss their illness with that parent.

Children also may inadvertently learn of the nature of their illness in a manner that *is* not supportive. If children find out their infection status from someone other than a parent, they may feel unable to confide in their parent or feel a need to conceal that they are aware of their diagnosis. Studies on the impact of HIV/AIDS disclosure to children are limited. Preliminary studies suggest, however, that children who know their HIV/AIDS status have higher self-esteem than infected children who are unaware of their status. Parents who have disclosed the status to their children experience less depression than those who do not. Disclosure should not only take into consideration of the child's age, maturity and the complexity of family dynamics, but clinical context as well. Children who are at their critical stage of illness, handling the consequence of illness, that may be death, rather than just the disclosure of disease may be more appropriate to address, at that stage. Although disclosure should occur in a supportive environment that optimally should include knowledgeable professionals and parents, some parents may decide to have professionals assume this responsibility. Ongoing counselling is required throughout the child's infection, which will be helpful in obtaining parental understanding of the importance of disclosure.

From the above analysis, it is clear that a considerable progress has been made in understanding the natural course of disclosure of HIV/AIDS status and its consequences among children. Infected children differ from infected adults in several ways. Firstly, the disease progresses much more rapidly in children; secondly, children have higher viral loads than those usually seen in adults; thirdly, children have recurrent invasive bacterial infections more often; and finally, opportunistic infections often present as primary diseases with a more aggressive course because of the lack of prior immunity. Despite these differences, children's cellular responses to HIV/AIDS are similar to those of adults and they respond almost as well to aggressive, multi-drug antiretroviral regimens.

The key to prevention of HIV/AIDS infection in children clearly lies in preventing their parents from acquiring the disease. Unfortunately, except for isolated successes such as in Uganda and Thailand (associated with sex education and increased condom use) (UNAIDS, 2000), there is little hope that the expansion of the pandemic will be halted soon. Much more efforts need to be directed at the socio-cultural and economic aspects of preventing the spread of HIV and linking them to the biomedical approaches.

According to Global AIDS and Health Fund,

"Tomorrow's children will judge our resolve or inaction."

Significant progress in women's rights has been made in India since independence. However, there is still a long way to go. Society continues to be structured in ways that favor men, the so-called stronger sex--as the earning power lies with men. In large part, this is due to society's prevailing assumptions about women's "natural" maternal or mothering tendencies. The segregation of men and women in the labor market leads to a considerable gap between men and women's income level, and this discrepancy in income, in turn, translates to differences in overall social value of men and women in a society that tends to place primary value on how much income a person generates (Ghodially and Kumar, 1998). But most women with HIV/AIDS are infected through heterosexual contact, injection drug use being the second leading exposure category for women.

The heterosexual exposure category suggests continuing gender inequality. Even in the 21st century, the notion that a woman's happiness and wholeness depend entirely on her affiliation with men remains a common perception.

According to a feminist poetess and essayist Adrienne Rich, we are still trained to think that women need men as *"social and economic protectors, for adult sexuality, and for psychological completion"*. And those women whose primary affiliation or attachment is not with men are perceived to be fundamentally abnormal or deviant. Simultaneously, society continues to perceive women as sexual objects for the control and consumption by men. The high rate of heterosexual transmission of HIV, thus, implicates the prevalence of traditional sexist thinking, fostering women's continued dependence on men and continues sexual objectification of women. Women who are highly dependent on men for social and economic support may find limitations in their ability to negotiate in heterosexual relationships. This has serious implications in terms of HIV prevention.

For male-dependent women, condom negotiation may not be feasible if women perceive that their male sexual partner(s) will respond negatively to the suggestion of condom use. As a result, these women may find that participation in unprotected sex is a better option than an estranged relationship.

One of the men, 36 years, HIV positive, stated,

> *"she has very less knowledge on all issues in life including on sex, HIV etc. so she better listen to me. As a male I meet more people, internet with the outside world. So I know what is right or wrong for her ..."*

Interestingly, a man aged 29 years, HIV positive, says,

> *"... my wife wants me to use condom --she says that's what the health worker told her--Health worker who is also a woman. I don't want to use condoms. My wife should accept me as I want to be ..."*

Another man aged 41 years, HIV positive, says,

> *". . . because of my HIV status, my wife threatens me often that she will leave me. But I know very well she is dependent on me financially. Being a woman I know she cannot survive alone economically or socially . . . ."*

The socially anticipated roles have placed women at risk for HIV. According to Carole Campbell, Professor at California State University, women may engage in unprotected sex with men to attain social status, fulfill emotional needs and achieve economic stability. Because women are commonly expected to negotiate issues inherent in sexual relationships (such as condom use by their male partners), the responsibility of HIV/AIDS prevention falls on women. But, this expectation ignores the fact that men and women do not have equal power in relationships. The expectation further ignores how, in India and its culture, we tend to celebrate and encourage displays of male virility through sexual acts. Placing the responsibility of HIV/ AIDS prevention on women, moreover, ignores the violence that is pervasive in Indian culture. It also ignores the existence of "compulsory heterosexuality", which is what Adrienne Rich defines as *"the ideology that demands heterosexuality"*. The need to openly display one's heterosexuality through participation in heterosexual sex, in other words, defines the very characteristic of compulsory heterosexuality. Most cultures, in the world, cast women as the primary caretakers and nurturers of men and children. As a result, women frequently sacrifice their own needs, including their health care needs.

The health needs of HIV-positive and HIV-at-risk women, then, are often subordinate to the needs of men. This, of course, may ultimately prove consequential to women's health. For HIV-positive women, HIV/AIDS is just one of many obstacles that they must contend with on a daily basis. But women with HIV/ AIDS nevertheless are expected to not only continue with their daily care-taking rituals of others, but also they are, to some degree, expected to cope with HIV/AIDS casually, as if it were a routine illness. Hence, in many respects, all those individuals who are in a woman's custody--that is, all those for whom she is responsible in terms of care taking --reap the benefits from her labor, but their benefits come at the expense of the woman's own health and general wellness. The HIV/ AIDS pandemic necessarily implicates gender. The increasing rates of heterosexual transmission of HIV/AIDS among women highlight profound gender inequality, illuminating the presence of culturally enforced attitudes and expectations that continue to perpetuate the subordinate status of women.

To prevent the spread of HIV/AIDS among women, we, as a society, must enable all men and women to have--regardless of person or situation --greater access to education, information and participation in all levels of the labor force. Education and greater earning power in turn are associated with both increased self-awareness (including a greater awareness of the injustice of social inequality) and autonomy characteristics that allow women not only to more effectively negotiate personal relationships but also to resist attempts to subjugate women physically, psychologically or in other respects.

Her Will: Need Consulate?

Social and cultural determinants relating to women's position in Indian society directly affect their ability to care for their health. This is especially so in regard to HIV/ AIDS. Women's dependency on men, their lower level of education, limited access to resources and lower economic status is enhanced in the area of health care, particularly in their incapacity to protect themselves from sexually-transmitted infection. Increasingly it is being recognized that cultural values and the status of women in a society are important aspects of HIV/AIDS pandemic. HIV/AIDS is a development and gender issue. Social inequality between men's and women's roles and positions is cited as being most responsible for the spread of HIV/AIDS in India.

Women tend to have limited knowledge of the problems and the risks associated with HIV/AIDS virus and also less social power to oppose risk conditions (see Chapter 5). That is, women's pre-existing social, economic, legal and political disadvantage heightens their vulnerability not only to risk of HIV/AIDS infection but also to most of the impact of the epidemic. This includes lack of social and physical access to health care services for women, which further increases their vulnerability to HIV/ AIDS.

In addition, female poverty, a feature of Indian society, often brings with it an increased risk of HIV/AIDS through restricted access not only to health information, but also health care services such as condom supplies and STD treatments. On the one hand, Indian society does not frown on a man/husband seeking sex outside marriage. On the other hand, often sex with one's wife is seen as a duty and held in special regard in a sexual context. Indeed, sexual desire or lust for flush is sometimes considered shameful. For this reason, the seeking of sexual pleasure outside marriage is condoned. Nevertheless, prohibitions against intercourse during the wife's menstruation or for yearlong periods after childbirth may be a further contributing factor to men seeking sex outside of marriage. This has an obvious bearing on HIV/AIDS transmission.

A reason for sex outside marriage may be, for husbands who work away from the home for lengthy periods are not expected to deny themselves pleasure and a 'little fun'. According to community based care and support project investigator, a considerable number of male migrant workers engage in sexual encounters with women other than their wives while working away from their homes. Upon their return these men re-commence sexual relations with their wives. Usually no precautions, for example, condom use, are taken either with the wives or with the other women. The wives are thus exposed to the risk of HIV/AIDS transmission. An interesting aspect of this situation is that

> *"when men are infected, their wives are suspected of infidelity; when women are infected, they are assumed to have had multiple partners",*
>
> .... according to Bledsoe.

There are several ways in which women can suffer from psychological stress, physical suffering and economic costs related to the HIV/AIDS. Women may experience fear and concern of being infected with the virus from their husbands or partners. This reflects that women have a few opportunities to demand or request that their partners practice safe sex.

Discussion with a woman aged 34, HIV positive, expressed serious concern over the fact that her husband, who is a long distance truck driver, may have the HIV virus and that she is unable to instigate measures of protection for herself. She fears not only that she will get AIDS, but that if she becomes ill her children may suffer as well, due to her inability to care and provide for them.

Women can be affected psychologically by HIV/AIDS

in their role of caregiver. When family members fall ill, it is women who provide the nursing care and in the case of illness or the breadwinner, it is women who usually take over as providers of basic needs for themselves and other family members. Such women may face the fear of the death of their husband, the fear of becoming infected and feeling helpless, mental stress over the physical and psychological burden of care, and a sense of despondency and failure about the future. In this way Indian women are further disadvantaged with regard to their ability to intervene and reduce their own risk of HIV/AIDS infection.

In sum, the above analyses reveal that women and children are at special risk of HIV/AIDS infection. Increasingly, recognition is being given to this fact that there is a synergistic relationship between STDs and HIV/AIDS, and socio-cultural factors. Overall, it reflects that women have a low level of knowledge concerning HIV/AIDS--but their ignorance and fear will not protect them from the potential tragedy of AIDS. Both government and private organizations are working to raise women's HIV/AIDS consciousness, and many uncoordinated efforts to provide accessible and acceptable services for STD care and education are being developed and implemented now. Nevertheless, these efforts will have limited impact on the epidemic as long as perceptual awareness and gender inequalities are not addressed. HIV/AIDS is not 'just' a health problem, but also one, which is inextricably linked to the social context, cultural values and economic relations, which determine the interaction between individuals and within society.

Perception Towards Prevention

According to PLHAs, there is a widespread perception that the authorities and other health care providers have no policy on providing care to those already infected. A number of interventions have occurred and the government has tried its best to cope with but so far PLHAs have not received any fruitful services as outcome. This reflects that achieving results on account of many efforts--political commitments, culture of open debate, involvement of families and reasonable access to care--are not that easy a task in our community. India as a nation is culturally trapped in London's Victorian Era with respect to attitudes towards sex. If sex, transmission of diseases and safe sex is taboo then no amount of intervention will improve the problem. One can blame easily the mass media, which is highly responsible and hides everything with respect to sex.

According to an investigator aged 40, HIV positive, about vulnerability

> *"Everything surrounds sickly Bollywood movies where pretty girls run around into their lovers arms with a song playing in the backgound. A dreamworld where the camera is "cut" where the couples kiss! I say this because the people in India can be reached by the Bollywood powers but this health issues like HIV/AIDS have not even been considered. Reaching people with health education intervention is impossible. To begin, people would probably never believe it nor would they attend. When it comes to sex on screen or even featuring important matters like condoms, this is rarely seen."*

This questions the credibility of India, which is the land of the "Kamasutra". Sexual experimentation is rife in all arenas. It's simply that warnings of the dangers are ignored due to the conservative attitude that sex should be kept behind closed doors. Hypocrisy is the worst enemy of Indian cultural setting. Facades are a great evil for those who place themselves in danger everyday. At the same time, the Indian media fails to educate people due to the attitude that *'sex must never be seen to happen'*. Quite frankly it does, despite various protests. If it didn't then, it is hardly believable that the entire population originates from the stork!! That is of course what Indians would like their younger generation to believe!

Husband told me about his HIV positive status before having intercourse with me--

> *"I wouldn't be suffering like this. And, I don't need to think about my daughter's HIV positive status, if he told me we are HIV positive."*
>
> .... says woman aged 37

She adds,

> *" We need to promote open discussion about the sex and HIV / AIDS. Every girl and woman must know what is sex and its consequences."*

This reflects that until India as a nation alter its attitudes towards (safe) sex to even bring themselves to publicize condoms on a regular basis, HIV/AIDS will continue to rise to uncontrollable levels. This requires timely advocacy urging the immediate upscaling of the efforts for preventing the transmission of HIV/AIDS in our community.

Bridging the Gaps

At present there is no cure for HIV/AIDS. Primary education about human behaviour and sexuality is appropriate for the adolescent development as an individual. If adolescents' minds are kept in dark, it can prove to be disastrous. Adolescents should be brought up in a curriculum that he/she gets accurate information about sex from teachers, parents as well as from the society. It is a de-facto that adolescents get to know about sex from unreliable sources and ill-informed peers. Sex education should be made an integral part of all learning/training centers' curriculum and taken up seriously. Critics are however concerned that introducing sex education in all learning/ 'training centers' curriculum might bring in perverted ideas in the minds of adolescents and lead them to an untoward thought process, but on the contrary they would get the right stuff, at the right time from the right source. So it is almost imperative that at the correct age, adolescents should be provided with interactive sex education in all learning/training centers'.

Evidentally, India is a society at war with its own beliefs and traditions. Gender inequality, economic discrimination and illiteracy are rife. HIV/AIDS will decimate India if its society fails to appreciate the need and urgency for change in a wider context within which risk occurs. At the same time, 'prevention is better than cure' needs to be taken a step further. Prevention alone has not worked in other infectious diseases unless it is taken up as a national/ global campaign, for example small pox or polio (which is still ongoing). No infectious disease could be controlled by prevention alone.

REFERENCES

Indrani, "The AIDS Epidemic and the Economic Burden of Treatment in India", Presented at the Meeting of the UNAIDS Reference Group on Economics. Cuernavaca, Mexico, February 2001.

Development in India", Background Study for the Swedish Country Strategy for India 2003-2007, Sida, New Delhi. 2003.

Indian Council of Medical Research (ICMR), 1988, "Changing trends in sero-surveillance for HIV infection". *ICMR Bulletin* 18: 39.

Jain K., *Tribal sex seller women and HIV/AIDS infection in India. Xth International conference on AIDS.* Yokohama, Japan, 1994.

Jana S., Bandyopadhyay N., Mukherjee S., Dutta N., Basu I., Saha A., "SID/HIV intervention with sex workers in West Bengal, India", *AIDS* 1998.

Kumar M.S., Mudaliar. S., Thayagarajan. S.P. Kumar S., Selvanayagam A., "Rapid assessment and response to injecting drug use in Madras, South India". *International Journal of Drug Policy.* 11. 1-2: pp 83-98. 2002.

MAP. *The status and trends of HIV/AIDS/STI epidemics in Asia and the Pacific.* October 4 2001. Melbourne. Australia.

National AIDS Control Organisation. *Combating HIV/AIDS in India. 2000-2001.* Ministry of Health and Family Welfare, National AIDS Control Organisation. Government of India.

National Family Health Survey -2 (1995-1999. International Institute of Population Sciences. Mumbai.

Panda S., Bijaya L., Devi, N.S., et al., "Interface between drug use and sex work in Manipur, *National Medical Journal of India* Vol. 14: No 4. 2001.

Ramasundaram S., "Can India avoid being devastated by HIV". *British Medical Journal,* 324: 182-183 (26 January). 2002.

Reid G., Costigan G., *Revisiting 'The Hidden Epidemic:' A Situation Assessment of Drug Use in Asia in the context of HIV/AIDS.* The Centre for Harm Reduction. The Burnet Institute, Australia. January 2002.

Salunke. S.R., Shaukat M., Hira S.K., Jagtap M.R., "HIV/AIDS in India: A country responds to a challenge". *AIDS.* 12 (Suppl B), 1998.

Suniti Solomon, et. al., "HIV in India". *Special Contribution.* Volume 10 Issue 3 July/August 2002.

Third International Conference on AIDS INDIA. Chennai, 'India. December 1-5. 2001.

Times of India, State orders HIV infection enquiry at blood banks. (Kolkata) 5 March, 2002.

UNAIDS, *Workplan- 1999-2001. A Strategic Response to the HIV epidemic by the government of India, the UN and its development partners in India.*

CHAPTER 3

Fighting HIV: Some Guidelines

Currently, the world over, it is estimated that over 33 million people are infected with HIV, and over 16 million have died of AIDS-related illnesses. In many resource-poor countries and among marginalised groups of people in industrialised countries, the number of new HIV infections continues to rise. In some countries in Africa, AIDS-related morbidity and mortality are causing major reversals in development, childhood mortality, and survival and life expectancy. Realisation of the enormous impact that HIV/AIDS is having on the well-being of individuals. families and communities, forced governments and communities to review the effectiveness of their HIV/AIDS programmes. In the context of such reviews, some governments have considered whether the principles of confidentiality and informed consent contribute to the spread of HIV.

There is concern that these principles allow a person who is HIV positive to keep his status confidential, and refuse to share it with sexual or drug-injecting partners, family members or the community. Governments and others have asked whether these principles hinder efforts to prevent the spread of HIV and deny protection to the sexual and drug-injecting partners of those infected. There is also concern that the principle of confidentiality contributes to the "invisible" status of the epidemic and to the general denial of HIV/AIDS within communities and nations. As a result, policymakers have begun to consider legislation and practice that would allow breaches in confidentiality, mandatory partner notification and named HIV case-reporting for public health reasons; and would permit the criminal prosecution of individuals who are considered to have spread the virus deliberately.

To address these concerns, and in response to a request for WHO assistance made by Ministers of Health in Africa, WHO (AFRO) and the UNAIDS Secretariat cosponsored a regional technical consultation on notification, confidentiality and HIV/ AIDS in August 1999 in Windhoek, Namibia.

A meeting statement was produced that aimed to assist Ministers of Health and other partners in southern Africa to develop policy and guidelines. Further, in October 1999, the UNAIDS Secretariat and WHO cohosted an international consultation in Geneva. Switzerland, on HIV reporting and disclosure. This consultation included epidemiologists, public health official national AIDS programme managers, people with HIV/AIDS lawyers and human rights activists from more than 20 countries. The Windhoek and Geneva meetings confirmed that the principles of confidentiality and informed consent do not contribute to the spread of HIV/AIDS. Indeed, if employed in the appropriate context and in creative and culturally sensitive ways, confidentiality and informed consent can help to decrease the spread of HIV/AIDS. Rather, responsibility lies with the denial, stigma and discrimination which continue to surround HIV/AIDS, and which result in a high level of secrecy concerning the epidemic. This denial, stigma and discrimination, and the resulting secrecy, must be overcome and the HIV/AIDS epidemic normalised into what it is -- a viral infection, as well as major human, health and development crisis. Relevance of ethical principles such as confidentiality and informed consent has been raised throughout the history of the response to the epidemic. That these come under examination, again at this stage is a necessary and welcome development. In general at highlights the need for greater efforts to 'open up' the HIV/ AIDS epidemic. In particular, it highlights the need to identify more clearly the causes and consequences of the denial, stigma, discrimination and secrecy that surround HIV/AIDS and hinder effective responses. The denial, stigma, discrimination and secrecy regarding HIV/AIDS continue to exist even though prevalence of HIV, and deaths from AIDS, are very high in many places. They stem from several causes.

Individually, people do not want to acknowledge that HIV/AIDS is within their communities, that it poses a real personal threat to them and to their families, that they themselves may already be infected and that they may be transmitting the virus to their sexual or drug-injecting partners. Furthermore, people do not want to get tested for HIV or to disclose their HIV status because they fear that they will be rejected by their partners, that they will face stigma and discrimination, and/or that they will be blamed for infecting others. Finally, most people in the developing world know they will not have access to drugs and treatment which would slow down the progression of the disease or alleviate its pain and suffering.

Thus, denial, stigma, discrimination and lack of access to care stem from, and lead to, a sense of fear and hopelessness, and encourage secrecy about HIV/AIDS. Collectively, many resource-poor communities are struggling with extremely difficult conditions in which to combat HIV/AIDS. They suffer from insufficient health care and education services, including insufficient voluntary testing and counselling; insufficient public education campaigns, particularly education targeted, to young people, women and marginalised groups; insufficient access not only to anti- retroviral drugs but also to drugs to reduce the pain and suffering caused by AIDS-related illnesses; and insufficient community organisation and support, including lack of a social and legal infrastructure to protect people from HIV-related discrimination. These conditions are exacerbated among marginalised groups in communities. These obstacles seriously hamper government and community efforts to prevent the spread of HIV and to provide care and support for those affected by HIV/AIDS. Governments and communities have felt at a loss to know how to combat this denial, stigma, discrimination and secrecy. This has justified calls for 'new or different' approaches to respond to the epidemic, particularly in high-prevalence areas Mandatory HIV case-reporting and disclosure of HIV status particularly to sexual partners but also to communities, have been suggested as sound public health measures. Discussions have been initiated nationally, regionally and internationally on how to:

(a) improve epidemiological surveillance of HIV and AIDS

(b) create greater openness about HIV/AIDS among individuals and within families and communities:

(c) better protect people not infected from becoming infected;

(d) encourage more people to test for HIV, inform sexual partners about the results and prevent further infections;

(e) increase acceptance, care and support for people and families affected by HIV/AIDS;

The UNAIDS Secretariat and WHO offer guidance concerning these issues in a context that involves commitment to human rights, ethical principles, public health and community empowerment.

Such a context protects the health and safety of the individual both infected and uninfected it also protects public health. It does so by creating an environment that encourages the most people to get tested for HIV encourages people to change their behaviour either to prevent their own infection or that of others and, where infected, to fectable and willing to disclose their status in a way that prevently onward transmission of HIV; and results in care and compassion. Such an environment will help to open up the epidemic; reduce the denial, stigma, discrimination and secrecy surrounding HIV/AIDS; and fashion programmes that allow governments, communities and individuals to deal with the causes and consequences of HIV/AIDS in the most effective and humane ways possible.

Confidentiality. i.e. retaining privacy, is an ethical principle particularly relevant in the provision of health care. The principle of confidentiality encompasses the view that a person should be entitled to privacy with regard to his or her most personal physical and psychological secrets; but it is also the basis for an effective relationship between patient/client and health care provider, and hence the basis for the effectiveness of many public health interventions which rest on these relationships. Only if a person feels sure that the health care provider will keep confidential any information provided will he come forward and share information that may be critical to making decisions about effective clinical care and treatment. Thus, health care professionals have long recognised and respected their duty, and the need, to protect the confidentiality of their patients.

Due to the need to protect confidentiality in order to provide effective health care, health care professionals also recognise that they should normally only disclose highly personal information, such as HIV status, with the informed consent of the patient. However, the principle of confidentiality is not absolute, and there are situations where it is not maintained. One of these occurs when necessary and relevant information is shared among health care professionals who are responsible for the clinical management of a person's health needs.

Often a small group of professionals, usually in a hospital or clinic setting, will share personal information about a client, including HIV status, which is essential to the effective treatment of the case, but confidentiality will be maintained within this professional group. Another situation where confidentiality may be breached without the consent of the patient occurs when there is a clear indication that a third party may be harmed by the actions of the patient. In these situations the ethical principle of confidentiality may conflict with the ethical principle to do no harm", and a difficult but necessary ethical weighing of the potential harms and benefits to the parties involved should be undertaken in order to decide how to proceed. The ethical principles of confidentiality and informed consent, which have private and public health benefits, should be distinguished from secrecy which is a state of affairs often resulting from fear, shame and/or a sense of vulnerability, Whether secrecy is maintained depends solely on the personal motives of those who hold the secret. Motives to maintain secrecy in the context of HIV/AIDS involve not only fear and shame, but also denial, and fear of rejection, stigma and discrimination. To the degree that secrecy harms the infected and the uninfected, and undermines an individual's family's or community's ability to cope positively with HIV/AIDS, it should be strongly combated. UNAIDS and WHO are of the view that the secrecy surrounding HIV/AIDS, and the related stigma, denial and discrimination, can best be countered by a greatly increased commitment to beneficial disclosure, ethical partner counselling and appropriate use of HIV case-reporting.

Survival Skills

Remarkably, providing survival skills is a vital part of HIV counselling Knowing about survival skills helps people accept a positive HIV test result because it reinforces the message that this result does not mean the end of their life. Survival skills should be discussed in all counseling sessions, including in sessions with clients who are unaware of their HIV status and are considering being tested. Counsellors need prepare for counselling sessions. There are, however, several things he can do to prepare himself.

He needs to find out as much information as possible about HIV, AIDS, and related subjects. This information should be accurate and uptodate. He has to make himself familiar with the skills needed to prolong life and the behaviors that speed up the progression of AIDS. If he knows other people dealing with similar problems for the client, explore the client's interest in meeting these people to help in the formation of support or self-help groups.

Begin to discuss survival skills with clients as early as possible, preferably during pre-test counselling. Most people going for an HIV test are already thinking about how a positive test result may affect their life. Knowing beforehand that there are survival strategies can ease the tension.

If the test does turn out to be positive, the knowledge that there is something one can do to stay healthy will help the client cope with receiving the result.

Some issues the counsellor should be aware of when he is counselling a person who intends to have an HIV test:

- Determine the reasons why the client has decided to have an HIV test. Sometimes people are pressured or coerced into having a test by another person such as a doctor, counsellor, or partner. It is important that the client, and nobody else, decides to have a test. Taking an HIV test is a big step and the client needs to be aware of the advantages and disadvantages. The test, should not be done without the client's full and genuine consent.
- Give the client accurate and uptodate information about HIV and AIDS, and correct any misconceptions the client might have. Give the client time to express any worries or fears, and address them before the test is taken.
- Stress the confidentiality of counselling and testing. It is important that the client understands that both the discussion and the results of the test will be confidential, and that nobody else will be told about them without the client's permission.
- If the client thinks that he or she might be HIV positive, you should explore the reasons. Help the

client assess the risks and the effects of HIV in preparation for the results.

- Whenever possible, help the client identify a support person -- a relative or a friend -- to provide company when going for the test results and for post-test counselling.
- If the client has a stable sexual partner, you should explain the advantages of getting tested and getting results with the partner. Explore the difficulties and possible consequences of disclosing the test results to the partner. Try to encourage the client to bring his or her partner to a pre-test counselling session.If the client has a stable sexual partner, you should explain the advantages of getting tested and getting results with the partner. Explore the difficulties and possible consequences of disclosing the test results to the partner. Try to encourage the client to bring his or her partner to a pre-test counselling session.
- If the client has a stable sexual partner, you should explain the advantages of getting tested and getting results with the partner. Explore the difficulties and possible consequences of disclosing the test results to the partner. Try to encourage the client to bring his or her partner to a pre-test counselling session.
- Prepare the client for both a positive and a negative HIV test result. In preparation for a negative result explore with the client how to reduce his or her personal risk for HIV infection. In preparation for a positive result introduce the subjects of survival skills and positive result that will be covered in much greater detail during post-test counselling.

Survival skills are a very important subject of post-test counselling. When people find out that they are HIV positive they often feel as if their world has fallen apart and that there is no point in living any longer. Post-test counselling should help people develop coping mechanisms for dealing with their HIV status, and to realise that life is not over just because of the result of a laboratory test.

Some issues the counsellor should be aware of when he is counselling persons who have returned for their HIV test result:

- Assure that the client is ready to receive the result. You can assume that most people who have returned to the testing centre want to know their test result, but you should still ask. If you sense some hesitation, talk about the reasons. The client may not be here out of his or her own free will. Discuss the advantages and disadvantages of knowing one's HIV status. Do not give the results until you are sure the client is ready to receive them.
- Assure the client again that the result of the HIV test and the discussions of the counselling session are confidential and will not be disclosed to anyone without his or her explicit permission.
- If and when the client is ready, give the test result.

If the counsellor have just give a positive HIV test result to a client:

- Observe and assess the client's emotional state. People react in different ways to a positive result. Some people show little emotion, others react with emotional outbursts. The counsellor's role is to assist clients to deal with their emotions as they are expressed.

- Address the client's needs and concerns. This discussion must be driven by the client and not by the counsellor. This means that you should respond to the issues and topics brought up by the client, but not tell the client how he or she is feeling or what emotions he or she might be going through.
- Find out if the client has had a pre-test counselling session and what was discussed. Sometimes people are tested for HIV without pre-test counselling. In this case, you should try and cover the most important pre-test issues in the post-test counselling session.
- Discuss survival skills and strategies for positive living. These include risk reduction, nutrition, and stress management.
- Disclosure of HIV status is a very important issue at the time of post-test counselling. Explore to what extent this has been discussed during pre-test counselling, has the client thought about whom to tell about the result? Who are the people that the client can rely on for support? Do not rush the client into making decisions about disclosure. This is a big step that has to be considered carefully.
- Remember that your main task when counselling a person who has just received a positive HIV test result is to provide emotional support and information. If you do not have the information, refer the client to another counseling or to another source of information or support.
- After receiving a positive HIV test result, many people find it hard to concentrate on specific issues. The client's mind is racing--many points covered in the counselling session will be quickly forgotten.

Encourage the client to return for further sessions of supportive counselling where issues can be dealt with, as they become important and relevant. Make a follow-up appointment.

Stress Management

Dealing with stress is an important survival skill. A person who is stressed may show the following signs and symptoms;

- social withdrawal, loss of interest in surroundings;
- moodiness, irritability, or intolerance;
- difficulty falling asleep, or early morning wakening;
- constant fatigue, difficulty in getting out of bed;
- upset stomach, loss of appetite, over-eating;
- headaches or pain in the neck and shoulders;
- loss of sexual desires or urges;
- loss of ability to concentrate;
- loss of interest in activities, apathy;
- poor performance at work or in school;
- pacing or restlessness;
- increased use of alcohol, tobacco, or other drugs.

A counsellor should help the clients to manage their stress:

- Encourage the clients to talk about the issues troubling them.
- Discuss potential sources of support. Sources of support can be found amongst family, relatives, friends, church groups, support groups, or counselling organisations.

- Encourage clients to rest, relax, and get enough sleep Some people find it relaxing to pray, meditate, or to talk to themselves in private. Physical exercise is very effective for stress management. Encourage clients to take up yoga, go jogging, join an aerobics class, or go dancing.
- Encourage clients to spend time with other people and help them identify people they feel secure with.
- Try to identify the problem. It is easier to deal with stress once you know what is causing it.
- Death or sickness in the family is a common cause of stress. Another booklet in this series provides counselling guidelines for palliative care and bereavement.
- People are affected differently by stress. After a stressful event some people "shut down" and adopt a life style of mere survival without joy or expectations. Others react by becoming over-active and pushing themselves harder.
- Encourage them to adopt techniques like affirmation (I am .... I can.... I will...) and relaxation (meditation, exercise) to help them return to a pace and a style of life that is comfortable for them..
- Remember that some stress can be positive. Knowing that they are HIV positive has motivated many people to plan their lives more carefully and deliberately. They are achieving much more because they have developed a positive attitude to life.

Possible causes of stress that are related to HIV infection may be:

- receiving the result of a positive HIV test;
- involuntary disclosure of a positive HIV test;
- break-up of family or of a relationship;
- death of a spouse or child;
- financial difficulties;
- loss of employment;
- inability to talk about one's problems;
- isolation due to expected or actual stigma;
- belief that death is imminent;
- fear of dying.

Beneficial Disclosure Support

In the context of HIV/AIDS, the term 'disclosure' refer to the act of informing any individual or organisation of the HIV status of an infected person, or it refers to the fact that such information has been transmitted, by any means, by the person him or herself, or by a third party with or without consent. However, the purposes and the consequences of disclosure may be beneficial or harmful. Examples of beneficial disclosure involve instances where an HIV-positive person informs a sexual partner of his status for prevention purposes, or informs family, community members or health care workers in order to share vital personal information and obtain support. Or disclosure may involve a health care worker providing information regarding an HIV/AIDS case on a confidential basis to other health care workers involved in the management of the patient: to a health authority for surveillance purposes: or, where necessary, to a partner of an HIV-positive person to prevent onward transmission of HIV.

Incidence of harmful disclosure involve cases where

disclosure is made without the consent of the person who is HIV positive and has adverse consequences for that person, such as stigma, abandonment, physical violence, imprison-ment, loss of job or housing, or other forms of discrimination. Harmful disclosure may also impair prevention and care activities. Where people fear forced testing, or disclosure involving lack of confidentiality, they will avoid HIV counselling, testing, treatment and support, because these are likely to mean that their HIV status will become known against their will and they will face stigma, discrimination, lack of privacy and other negative effects. Thus, fear of lack of confidentiality and forced disclosure drives people away from HIV services, reducing opportunities to encourage and empower people to change their behaviour in order either to avoid getting infected or to avoid passing on their infection.

It may also drive people away from other health care services, such as antenatal care or blood donation. Beneficial disclosure is voluntary; respects the autonomy and dignity of the affected individuals; maintains confidentiality as appropriate; leads to beneficial results for those individuals, and for their families and sexual and drug-injecting partners; leads to greater openness in the community about HIV/AIDS; and meets the ethical imperatives of the situation where there is need to prevent onward transmission of HIV.

Such beneficial disclosure, with its elements of voluntariness and confidentiality, not only maintains ethical principles but also serves a direct public health function, because it encourages people to access HIV prevention and care services. It does this by establishing a climate of trust between health care providers and those who need HIV services, allaying their fears and respecting them as people who can and will make the right decisions regarding their behaviour.

Beneficial disclosure also serves the goal of opening up the HIV/AIDS epidemic. As more people feel able and willing to disclose their status, there grows a critical mass of individuals and families within a community, and indeed within a nation, who are openly involved in dealing with the epidemic in positive and supportive ways.

As a consequence, discrimi-nation, stigma and secrecy are reduced. Nevertheless, preconditions are necessary to promote beneficial disclosure and to encourage people to access prevention and care programmes. People must have access to voluntary counselling and testing (VCT) services in which they can learn their HIV status and receive support and referral in dealing with the news. Furthermore, they must have an incentive to find out their status such that it will mean greater social support, access to health care options and an increased ability to live a rewarding life regardless of a negative or positive status. Up to 90 per cent of HIV-positive people in low-income countries do not know their HIV status due to the fact that there are few VCT facilities available to the population most affected by HIV/AIDS. Even where testing is available, many people do not want to be tested because of a perception that 'nothing is to be gained' by knowing an HIV-positive status. For the poor there will be little access to HIV/AIDS treatment and care.

Furthermore, there will likely be stigma and discrimination to be faced if found to be HIV positive. However, even in resource-poor settings much can be done to improve access to voluntary counselling, HIV testing, treatment and care, though this may involve a shift of resources from "traditional" HIV programmes and activities.

Primarily, there must be greater investment in establishing VCT services in communities. Secondly, incentives must be created to encourage people to undergo testing. These should take the form of community services providing support, treatment and care.

Finally, disincentives to test, such as stigma and discrimination, should be removed. There are insufficient VCT services in the communities most in need of them. More resources from national AIDS programmes should be devoted to establishing such services, which can take many forms. Most important are that VCT services are integrated into existing services where applicable (e.g. antenatal care, sexually transmitted infection (STI) clinics, family health clinics); they are user friendly (particularly to youth and women); are accessible to marginalised groups (e.g.. the poor, rural populations, sex workers, drug injectors, migrants); and are designed to tie the individual using them into other support and care options (e.g., referral to STI services, support groups, family outreach programmes).

The creation and availability of such services is a prerequisite if people are to learn about their HIV status and find ways of dealing with it constructively, including through disclosure. However, the existence of VCT services is not in itself enough to get people to come forward for HIV testing. There must be incentives, and these should take the form of greater availability and affordability of care, treatment and support. In resource-poor settings, treatment, in the form of drugs, and care options are very limited. However, these obstacles can in part be overcome by innovative and far-reaching community-based programmes.

Such programmes offer outreach to affected families, voluntary and confidential counselling and testing, support groups, home visits, follow-up and involvement of people living with HIV/AIDS in prevention and care activities. They may also offer models of how to 'live positively' with HIV/ AIDS, through which people maximise their personal and social resources, live as best as possible in the present and plan realistically for the future.

Examples of such effective community-based programmes can be found in Uganda, Tanzania and Thailand, where campaigns by non-governmental organisations (NGOs) to encourage testing have created more openness and discussion about HIV. In the parts of these countries where HIV testing has been made reasonably accessible to affected communities, the synergistic link between reducing stigma, increasing voluntary testing and encouraging disclosure has been confirmed.

Each of these activities reinforces the others and leads to greater numbers of people taking advantage of voluntary counselling, testing and support. This leads to more voluntary disclosure (to spouses, lovers, family members, friends and health care providers), the adoption of low-risk behaviour and a movement towards positive living. When such programmes are well integrated into the community and are responding to its needs, they can have a profound influence on how HIV/AIDS is perceived at the individual, family and community levels.

Positive-living models, as well as the active involvement of people living with and affected by HIV/AIDS, help to change attitudes from stigma and discrimination to respect and support. Affected families and communities are able to embrace their situation, are given support in how to best deal with it, while the family member who is HIV positive is still able to contribute to family and community efforts. This helps to reduce the stigma and to change public perceptions of HIV and people living with HIV/AIDS.

It also helps to encourage more people who do not know their status to come forward voluntarily for counselling and testing. Thus, greater investment needs in creating the facilities for HIV testing, as well as in backing community-based programmes which create a supportive environment and encourage people to come forward for HIV testing, counselling, care, treatment and support. Due to considerable shame, secrecy and fear surrounding HIV, people infected with HIV are highly stigmatised. HIV is also the cause of human rights violations and acts of discrimination.

As a result of the stigma and discrimination surrounding HIV/AIDS, those who do know their HIV status are afraid to disclose it because of the risk of job loss, social ostracism, violence and threats to their lives, and other adverse consequences. Those who do not know their status are afraid to get tested if they fear that the results will be made known against their will and they will face stigma and discrimination. Thus, to encourage voluntary testing, beneficial disclosure and use of HIV services, the disincentives of stigma and discrimination, and lack of confidentiality, must be removed. Many steps can be taken to reduce stigma and discrimination. One of the most under-utilised has been public information campaigns which focus specifically on the promotion of tolerance, compassion and non-discrimination. Though the world has been inundated with public information about the fact that HIV cannot be transmitted casually, this information has not done enough to alleviate fear of HIV and AIDS and of people living with them.

Public information campaigns should be conducted

which involve creative, attractive, powerful messages against discrimination and stigma. Public forums on HIV/AIDS and/or community discussion groups, which focus on compassion, tolerance and support, should also be held. Where there is protection against violence and discrimination, public figures, including those living with HIV, should be involved in these public campaigns. The involvement of people living with HIV/AIDS in public campaigns, and in policy, programmatic and community activities, is critical to give a human face to the epidemic, to reaffirm the value of people with HIV/AIDS and to change attitudes of stigma.

It also ensures that policies and programmes will be sensitive to the actual needs and realities of those affected by HIV/AIDS. Other measures can be undertaken at a national level, such as the enactment of laws and policies against HIV-related discrimination and against breaches in confidentiality and informed consent.

The training and sensitisation of professionals who work with people affected by HIV/AIDS in one essential step. It is often at the hands of such professionals that people affected by HIV/AIDS suffer the worst discrimination, despite the professional and ethical responsibility to, treat people who are HIV positive with dignity and compassion, and to protect their confidentiality in appropriate ways. Key professionals who might benefit from training in nondiscrimination, confidentiality and informed consent are health care workers, police, social service providers, lawyers and judges. Health care workers should be more empowered to handle the medical, as well as psychosocial, management of clients with HIV/AIDS.

This should include training and empowerment regarding universal precautions against transmission of infectious diseases, as it is the fear of transmission of HIV among health care workers that often leads to stigma and discrimination against people with HIV/AIDS. Experience has shown that the impact of this training in health settings needs regular monitoring and staff updating to ensure that infections control procedures are maintained.

For enthusing beneficial disclosure, UNAIDS and WHO recommend the following:

(b) Encourage participation of people living with HIV/AID in public information campaigns and in HIV programmes and policy formulation.

(a) Conduct public information campaigns and community forums aimed at promoting tolerance, compassion and understanding, and reducing fear, stigma and discrimination.

(c) Establish more VCT services, including in rural areas and for marginalised groups.

(d) Support governmental agencies. NGOs and community based organisations (CBOs) to make community-based services, including VCT, family outreach, community support, positive living, support groups and care options more widely available.

(e) Encourage the media to report on HIV/AID in a responsible, non-discriminatory and non-sensational manner.

(f) Train health care workers in the management of HIV and universal precautions, in attitudes of non-discrimination, acceptance and compassion, and in the principles of confidentiality and informed consent.

(g) Train other professionals (social workers, police, lawyers, judges) in attitudes of non-discrimination, acceptance and compassion, and in the principles of confidentiality and informed consent.

(h) Create legal support services for those who have suffered discrimination based on HIV status.

(i) Enact or reform laws, administrative guidelines and professional codes of conduct to prohibit discrimi-nation and breaches of confidentiality related to HIV status.

(j) Train key personnel in non-health employment settings, including human resource management in industry, in promoting non-discriminatory practices in the workplace.

Remarkably, the counsellor should be aware of the following disclosure issues when counselling for survival skills:

(a) The respondents, whom clients want to disclose their HIV status to, should have correct information about HIV and AIDS, and should have an open and non-stigmatising attitude towards people living with HIV. You may need to help some clients prepare their respondents.

(b) People who plan to disclose their HIV status need a lot of support and emotional preparation.

(c) Talking to somebody who is HIV positive may be very helpful to a person who is considering disclosure. Some support groups of people living with HIV have trained volunteer counsellors. They have personal experience of sharing information about their HIV status and can give guidance to the client. Joining a support group and talking to other people living with HIV is always a good idea, and it is particularly helpful for reaching a decision on disclosure.

(d) Some clients may ask for your presence when disclosing their HIV status. The presence of a counsellor can support both the client and the confidante. Remember that finding out that a loved one is infected with HIV can be very stressful.

(e) People should never he forced or pressured to disclose their HIV status: they must only do so when they feel ready to deal with the consequences. The client and not the counsellor has to decide whom to toll and when. This may he difficult for the counsellor who may know the client's family or sexual partner.

(f) Encourage the clients to be selective about disclosure. There are advantages and disadvantages to disclosure in each situation.

Treatment and Medicines

There are at least 15 different types of medicines known as antiretroviral drugs (ARVs). None of these drugs can cure AIDS or eliminate HIV, but if taken in the right combination, they can slow down the progression from HIV infection to AIDS Until recently, the drugs have been very expensive. However an intensive international lobby has resulted in the reduction of price in some countries, and the movement is gaining ground all over Africa. ARVs are already available in specialised clinics and big hospitals in all major cities, however still at a price that places them out of reach of most of the population. The currently available ARVs have to be taken for life. An effective treatment requires that at least three different drugs are taken at the same time. The drugs have major and sometimes life-threatening side-effects. In countries where these drugs have been available for a long time, about one in three persons stops taking them because of side effects or inability to follow the very strict drug regimen.

There are a number of other medicines that are known to beneficial to people living with HIV through their action of preventing common opportunistic infections. These are generally much more affordable and more widely available than ARVs. A counsellor should be aware of the types of medical treatment available to people living with HIV in the community, and how to access these treatments. However it is not wise to discuss medical therapies with the client unless expertise in this area. There are, however, alternate therapies being explored by PLWHA groups all over the world, whether they have access to ARV treatment or not. Many of these therapies have proven beneficial. The counsellor should explore among local support groups what types of natural or alternative medicines are available. The main guidelines in recommending alternative therapies are that the counsellor should not believe any claims of a "cure" of AIDS: the treatment should not do any harm to the patient: and it should not waste the patient's money without providing any benefit. Taking vitamin supplements, improved nutrition, prevention and early treatment of minor infections and avoiding stress can help prolong the client's life. Prompt attention to minor aches, pains, skin rashes, or injuries is essential for health and survival.

We are giving here, are some alternative therapies that PLWHAs have found useful. Remember that therapies such as aromatherapy, herbal remedies, reflexology, and hypnotherapy require a qualified practitioner:

meditation	the process of relaxing daily in a quiet setting to focus deeply on body energy and breathing techniques,
massage	kneading or rubbing parts of the body to promote circulation, suppleness, pain relief or relaxation,
relaxation	taking a short break away from work or chores to rest and control your breathing and body's response to increased tension,
aromatherapy	the application of fragrant essential oils to relieve tension and certain minor ailments,
reflexology:	a form of therapy Where pressure is applied to specific areas on the feet and hands, which stimulate the blood supply and nerves; to create a relaxing and healing effect on other body parts,
art therapy	drawing, painting or other forms of art as a way of relaxing or expressing emotions,
herbal remedies	the treatment of ailments with plants. There are many effective and widely known herbal remedies for common ailments such as diarrhoea. Some herbal remedies, for instance the African potato, are believed to boost the immune system and help fight off infections,
hypnotherapy	inducing a state of deep relaxation and concentration in which deeper parts of the mind are accessible for the treatment of emotional problems,
	Remind the client to "listen to your body" If eating in a certain way or receiving a certain type of treatment makes the client feel better, it will almost certainly be beneficial,

Keeping Fit Through Good Nutrition

Good nutrition is the only form of therapy that is available to most people. It is generally affordable because unrefined and unprocessed foods tend to be cheaper, though healthier. Nutrition as a therapy can improve the quality of life for people living with HIV because it can help them feel in charge. It allows them to do something practical to help themselves. People living with HIV need to protect their immune system because it is weakened by the HIV infection. They can do this by paying attention to two rules:

(i) Do not give your immune system other things to fight. You are most vulnerable to the effects of HIV when your body is trying to fight off other types of infections or when it is weakened by stress or exhaustion.

(ii) Strengthen your immune system by providing your body with the necessary nutrients to remain strong. This means eating a healthy and balanced diet.

A counsellor should become familiar with the rules for healthy eating in order to advise the clients.

When foods are "refined" it means that all the goodness has been removed. When foods have been "processed" it means things like colorings and preservatives—which can be harmful to the health—have been added.

A healthy diet should look like this:

(i) *Whole Grain (50%):* Grains should be whole, even if ground for thick porridge. For example, sorghum, millet, whole ground maize, whole wheat bread made from whole wheat flour, brown (unpolished) rice, barley, oat porridge, brekweet, or maltabella.

(ii) *Pulses (75%):* Pulses should make up the majority of protein in the diet: lentils, peas, nuts, dry bears, peanut, butter, chick peas, beans, and soya (soya mince or TVP) Soya and round nuts are "perfect proteins." Just like meat all the others must be combined with whole grains to make 100% protein.

(iii) *Vegetables (30%):* Combine yellow (pumpkin,

butternut, carrots, and sweet potato) with white (onions, leeks, cabbage, cauliflower) and green vegetables (spinach, rape, broccoli, okra, pumpkin leaves). Eat lots of vegetables everyday.

(iv) *Side Dish* (5%): This group should make up no more than 5 per cent of the total amount eaten. It includes:

fruits: eat when fresh and when in season. Avocados tomatoes and peppers are also in this group.

meat: little or no meat is recommended. Fish and-chicken are best. If meat is desired, eat liver, kidney or heart as they are high in iron.

dairy: milk, cheese and milk products should be eaten; very sparingly. Don't eat any dairy at all when you have diarrhoea, except yoghurt and lacto, which are good at all times. Eggs are good occasionally.

Vitamins and minerals are natural substances contained in food which are needed by the body in very small quantities for many different functions, including boosting the immune system. They are called micro-nutrients.

Many people living with HIV take additional micro nutrients in the form of tablets. But remember, vitamin tablets are no replacement for a healthy diet. If the client is poor do not recommend spending money on vitamin preparations. The priority should be a balanced nutrition for the family. If there is money left over, then the client may consider vitamin supplements.

One combination recommended by PLWHA groups consists of zinc, vitamins A, C, and E and selenium (ZACES).

ZACES is an infection fighting combination of vitamins and minerals. It increases the body's natural resistance and protects against the side effects of medications.

Zinc	1 x 10 mg tablet, twice daily
Vitamin A	1 x 25.000 I.U. tablet, once daily
'Vitamin C	2 x 500mg tablet twice daily (or 4 x 250mg twice daily
Selenium	1 x l00mg tablet daily (or 2 x 50 mg twice daily
Medox	12x12 1 tablet daily
Garlic	Up to 5 cloves a day

Foods to avoid include:

(i) Sugar and all foods containing sugar this includes cold drinks, cakes, sweets and cookies.

(ii) Tinned, processed and refined foods.

(iii) *Strong tea and coffee:* rooibos tea herb tea. fruit tea, bush tea and decaffeinated coffee can be good substitutes.

(iv) Alcohol and tobacco.

(v) *Red meat and pork:* liver and kidney are best if you crave red meat.

(vi) *Cooking oil:* except olive oil or cold pressed oils. Heating oil to cook with it destroys any goodness. Use it for salads only. Fats (dairy products) should be used sparingly and not at all when you have diarrhoea.

Health to achieve long-term survival with HIV can be compared to a table with four legs representing mental, physical, spiritual, and social health. The top of the table is nutrition.

(i) *Mental:* Encourage the clients to learn to co-exist with the virus. By giving the clients accurate and positive information about HIV and the immune system, you can help them adapt their lifestyle to overcome the immediate threats of HIV infection and to adopt a mental state in which they are not always feeling fragile and in danger.

(ii) *Spiritual:* Encourage the clients to seek spiritual support whatever their religious and cultural background. Prayer or meditation can induce deep mental and spiritual relaxation and renewal.

(iii) *Physical:* Encourage the clients to learn the practical steps they can take to improve and maintain health, e.g., exercising.

(iv) *Social:* Encourage the clients to join a support group and to become active in the community. Social isolation because of fear of being rejected or because of past experiences of rejection is bad for the clients' health and survival.

Sexual Health Maintenance

After receiving the result of a positive HIV test, some people feel off sex, some feel dirty or 'contaminated', and some believe that they can no longer have normal sexual relations. Yet a person living with HIV has the same sexual feelings and needs as anyone else, and there is no reason why these should be denied. Counsellors can help people understand this. At same time they must make their clients aware of the risks so they can make informed and responsible choices about sexual and reproductive lives.

The counsellor should be able to talk to the clients freely and objectively about sex. Condom use is a key issue to be discussed. The counsellor have to impress on his clients that consistent use of a male or female condom in every act of sexual intercourse is important for their own health and the health of their partners. If the partner is not infected, then he or she risks becoming infected with HIV. If the partner is already HIV positive, then both partners risk re-infecting each other and thereby increasing the number of virus particles in their system. This may result in a faster progression of the HIV infection to AIDS. Therefore, strict condom use or practising non-penetrative sex will protect both partners, whatever their status. Other important counselling issues related to reproductive and sexual health include:

(i) family planning;
(ii) abstinence;
(iii) partner notification;
(iv) sexually transmitted diseases;
(v) changes in the menstrual cycle;
(vi) transmission of HIV from mother to child.

Role of a counsellor is to:

(i) provide accurate and relevant information so that the client can make informed choices:
(ii) give and explore options: recognise and respect the uniqueness of the client: be aware of one's own beliefs and values;
(iii) know when to refer the client to another counsellor or agency for more appropriate and accurate information.

The clients may be concerned about whether or not they can have children. The counsellor need to advise them on the risks of HIV transmission to the child. Most of the transmission occurs during labour or through breast-feeding. However, most children born to HIV positive mothers are not infected with HIV, and there are interventions that can reduce the risk of HIV transmission to the infant. HIV positive women who wish to conceive should seek out good ante-natal and obstetric care. After delivery, they should avoid breast-feeding or practise "safer breast-feeding". The four components of safer breast-feeding are:

(i) exclusive breast-feeding for up to six months:
(ii) condom use during the lactation period;
(iii) immediate medical attention for minor infections of the breast or lesions in the baby's mouth;.and
(iv) proper positioning and attachment of the baby during every feed.

PROMOTING HIV CASE-REPORTING

HIV case-reporting has been promoted as a means to open up the HIV/AIDS epidemic: decrease denial improve access to prevention and care services for those affected by HIV/AIDS; and obtain more accurate information on the prevalence and incidence of HIV and AIDS for surveillance purposes. Under such a policy, health care providers would be required to report by name all HIV cases diagnosed by their, to a health authority. Other forms of case-reporting involve the use of a code, sometimes called a "unique identifier", for each case: or provide information on cases anonymously. While AIDS case-reporting has been implemented in most countries, implementation of HIV case-reporting has been much more limited. Many countries started to collect information on HIV cases at the beginning of the epidemic but later dropped the practice when the infection became widespread. The reasons were the high cost and complexity of maintaining the system, the lack of effective treatment or preventive options once people were discovered to be HIV positive, and the small additional benefit for surveillance purposes.

Notably, there has been a recent trend in high-income countries to employ HIV, as well as AIDS, case-reporting. This trend is based on the fact that, where antiretroviral therapies are available, the access to, and use of these drugs has dramatically decreased the incidence of AIDS. As a result, AIDS cases are no longer an accurate base for calculating back to HIV incidence and prevalence. Furthermore, in these countries, case-reporting of HIV helps to monitor the access of those who are HIV positive to appropriate services and treatment including the use of anti-retrovirals. However, neither the reporting of HIV cases nor the reporting of AIDS casts has been useful in low-income countries. For surveillance purposes, data collected on the basis of case-reporting of HIV or AIDS have been problematic.

Generally, HIV/AIDS surveillance involves the routine collection, analysis and dissemination of accurate epidemiological information regarding the spread and distribution of *HIV* infection. Surveillance is an essential part of the response to the epidemic entailing a number of important objectives:

(i) to monitor trends in prevalence and incidence of HIV in populations:

(ii) to assess disease burden in terms of morbidity and mortality due to HIV/AIDS:

(iii) to be able to plan HIV prevention and care programmes directed at the particular epidemiological situation:

(iv) to provide data for estimates and projections of the number of people with HIV/AIDS and AIDS-related mortality;

(v) to monitor the impact of the national response to the HIV AIDS epidemic:

(vi) to reinforce commitment to AIDS prevention and care through awareness of the numbers affected and their needs.

But the data obtained from HIV and AIDS case-reporting in many countries have not been useful for the stated objectives of surveillance largely for the following reasons.

(i) Less than 10 per cent of HIV-positive people have been tested for HIV, so most are unaware of their status.

(ii) Many people do not want to know their status, given the stigma and discrimination attached to a positive result and the fact that they will not have access to treatment or care.

(iii) Among health care providers, there are problems with under-diagnosis and underreporting of HIV and AIDS cases, including the fact that health care providers may be reluctant to report cases by name for reasons of confidentiality and privacy.

(iv) In contrast, where the information is provided ..anonymously to avoid breaches in confidentiality, there is potential for multiple reporting of the same case. There is insufficient capacity and infrastructure to maintain confidentiality for either named or coded reporting, which further deters people presenting for tests. These conditions make HIV case-reporting in resource-poor countries unreliable.

Advocates of HIV case-reporting point to potential benefits in terms of prevention and increased access to care. However, reporting HIV cases to health authorities does not necessarily lead to any additional benefit for either the client or the community, and may divert resources from more effective prevention and care strategies. Thus, where resources are limited, the appropriate balance must be found in the use of various prevention and care strategies that have different levels of costs and impact.

Strategies such as public information campaigns, youth education and distribution of condoms are relatively cost effective ways of reaching large numbers of people for prevention and care purposes. Case-reporting, however is expensive, and does not increase access to prevention and care services in itself.

To be effective in prevention and care terms case-reporting must be meaningfully integrated into a host of HIV-related services, such as VCT, health and social support services for those HIV positive and/or presenting with AIDS related illnesses, and greater access to HIV-related drugs and treatments.

Resources should be put into developing these services before they are significantly diverted to case-reporting

In light of these concerns, UNAIDS and WHO recommend HIV case-reporting only where certain conditions exist. These are:

(i) widespread access to, and use of HIV testing:

(ii) protection against breaches of confidentiality so as not to deter testing and reporting;

(iii) access to effective care, including anti-retrovirals;

(iv) capacity within the health system to collect accurate data, and to compile, analyse, and act upon them, including follow-up of cases.

Peer Counselling

Peer counselling overcomes barriers caused by class, age gender, sexual orientation, or HIV status. Peer counsellors have similar characteristics and experiences as their clients.

In peer counselling it is important to remember the following:

Do	*Do Not*
establish ground rules	judge or penalise
respect individuality acknow-	take over the burden
ledge the limitations of counsellors	argue
refer when stuck	ignore
listen	instruct

The advantages of peer counselling are that:

(i) it is easier for the client to feel at ease with a counsellor and the discussion will therefore he more open and free;

(ii) most barriers and boundaries between counsellor and client are removed, e.g., language, age gender etc. the sessions are informal and tend to be more spontaneous;

(iii) the counsellor and the client frequent the same social circles and often live or work in proximity. This makes the counselling sessions more accessible and often more affordable for the client;

(iv) the peer counsellor may provide a role model for the client that is easy to emulate: counselling may be linked to group support if several peers meet together.

Supportive Counselling

Supportive counselling may be centre-based--the client coming to see the counsellor when they need advice and support. Or it may be home-based. The advantage of home-based supportive counselling is that clients may be seen in their own environment.

It may not be very expensive if it is well planned, because several clients can often be seen in one visit. It is an opportunity to get to know clients better, to know their social and material situation, and to get to know their families and support networks. Examples of supportive counselling activities include:

(i) setting up tasks or goals (remember to check or follow up on goals on next visit or session);

(ii) providing a "sounding board" (being a listener) for clients to express their concerns or talk about particular issues;

(iii) working with the family, e.g., to improve the client's social support, or to help create more openness within the family;

(iv) helping clients to improve their communication skills, especially if they are preparing to disclose their HIV status.

There are limitations to remember:

(i) Supportive home-based counselling requires a lot of resources.

(ii) A long-lasting supportive counselling relationship may create material and emotional dependency on the counsellor.

(iii) Some clients may feel that their privacy is being invaded by the counsellor.

(iv) A counsellor may become too involved with a small number of clients, which will reduce overall effectiveness in job.

(v) Supportive counselling often involves repetition of things that have been discussed before. Clients who are stressed or upset will not absorb information the first time they hear it because of their emotional state. Be patient and be prepared to repeat discussions and to restate important messages several times.

II

PREVENTION AND CONTROL

Acquired Immune Deficiency Syndrome (AIDS) is a life, threatening condition caused by the Human Immune-deficiency Virus (HIV). Till today, there is no vaccine to protect the community from this dreadful virus. In 1981, researchers have identified two serotypes of HIV. HIV-1 is the predominant serotype worldwide. Eleven subtypes of HIV have been identified. In India, HIV-1 subtype C is the commonest. HIV-2 occurs most commonly in West Africa. Both HIV-1 and HIV-2 cause AIDS and the routes of transmission are the same. However, HIV-2 transmission is slightly less easy and HIV-2 may cause slower progression to AIDS. Today, HIV is prevalent in all parts of the world and has spread from urban to rural areas, and from individuals practising high risk behaviours to the general population.

More and more women attending antenatal clinics are testing HIV-positive, thereby increasing the chances of perinatal transmission. During sexual intercourse, damage to the lining of sexual organs facilitates transmission of HIV from the infected partner to the uninfected one by exchange of body fluids. It is easier for the virus to be transmitted if the uninfected partner is already suffering from some sexually transmitted disease/ reproductive tract infections, as in this case the lining of the organ is already compromised. The risk of HIV transmission through sharing of needles and syringes by injecting drug users (IDUs), on the other hand is very high. This is because blood is commonly sucked back into the syringe and then re-injected. The risk of HIV from mother to child transmission is believed to be 20-40 per cent in utero, during delivery and after birth. During the post-natal period, transmission of HIV infection from mother to child can occur through breast milk. It is recommended that all HIV mothers should be given an informed choice regarding the advantages and disadvantages of breast-feeding and safer alternatives to breast-feeding. Prevention is indisputably the most important objective as no curative drug is universally effective and no affordable prevention vaccine is likely to be available in, nor accessible to developing countries in the-foreseeable future.

Health education and behaviour modification is the prime focus of action for interrupting transmission. It is therefore important to have an information and education programme for all men and women, including adolescents, especially aimed at those who are at greater risk of HIV infection. It is also important to have facilities for detection and treatment of other sexually transmitted infections and to encourage an environment that promotes free and frank dissemination of information without stigmatisation and discrimination against suspected / known cases of HIV/AIDS. Prevention has maximum impact as part of comprehensive interventions, spearheaded by governments that break the silence around HIV/AIDS and deploy sufficient human and financial resources. Their impact is amplified by wider public health and development strategies addressing the underlying socioeconomic causes that leave people vulnerable to infection, as well as vulnerabilities arising from gender inequities, the denial of human rights and discrimination against marginalised groups.

Prevention efforts must be buttressed by well-supported community responses that include people living with HIV/AIDS, religious groups, and traditional and trusted leaders. And, in the context of more effective HIV treatment and the drop in anti-retroviral drug prices, prevention must be linked to the provision of care and support. As the epidemic is constantly shifting, prevention efforts must be tailored to developments in the epidemic, on the research front, and to evaluations that confirm success or failure. Like society itself, the epidemic is in constant flux as it adapts to surrounding factors and circumstances. The success stories of Cambodia, Senegal, Thailand, Uganda and urban Zambia, as well as those of a number of high-income countries, show that comprehensive prevention approaches are effective. These experiences provide clear evidence of what works:

- *Knowledge is not enough.* Behavioural change

requires locally-appropriate, targeted information, training in negotiating and decision-making skills, social and legal support for safer behaviours, access to the means of prevention (e.g., condoms or clean needles) and motivation to change behaviour.

- *The distribution of risk and vulnerability in societies varies greatly, as does the ability to locate and work with specific vulnerable populations.* No single prevention approach can be effective everywhere. To effectively produce and sustain behavioural change on a national scale, focused prevention programmes will involve multiple components, developed with the close input of each targeted population, to address the specific needs of vulnerable groups and the many factors influencing behavioural change.
- *Half-measures bring, at best, partial results.* Interventions that do not achieve sufficient coverage will simply fail to have a significant impact.
- *General population efforts are important, especially for the young.* Effective national programmes take into account the need to raise the awareness, knowledge, and HIV prevention and care skills among the rest of the population, especially the young, among whom almost half of all HIV transmission occurs.
- *Political leadership is essential to an effective response.* Political leadership and action are clearly needed to set the direction for a national response and initiate the development of policies that determine the strategy for managing the epidemic.
- *Partnerships are essential for effective prevention.* Since multiple programmes in multiple populations

are needed, it is crucial to create partnerships between different players, including people with HIV/AIDS.

Prevention depends on an environment of openness and inclusion that enables all people, including those living on the margins of society, to undergo voluntary testing, seek and receive treatment, alter their own behaviour, and become allies in the fight against HIV/AIDS. Successful responses challenge stigma and discrimination, protect the rights of those infected and affected by HIV, and include marginalised groups as active participants rather than mere 'beneficiaries' of services. Prevention efforts have always been hard to implement when access to treatment, care and support is limited. Without the hope of treatment, care and support, and fearing stigma and discrimination, people see little reason to learn about, or disclose, their HIV status.

Prevention is enhanced when it is linked to care and support. People are encouraged to come forward and get tested for HIV if they know treatment will be available. For those who test HIV-positive, treatment, care and support not only improve their quality of life, they also decrease the spread of infectious diseases through early diagnosis and treatment. Voluntary counselling and testing services are an entry point for behavioural change: they offer an opportunity for people worried about their serostatus to talk with medical and other trained staff, and discuss how they might prevent further spread of the infection. Open and compassionate care for HIV-infected people helps counter wider societal fears about HIV/AIDS. Ironically, in some high-income countries where access to treatment and care is widespread, prevention has increasingly become divorced from care. The result has been upturns in risky behaviour and, in some instances, increases in the number of new HIV infections. In such situations, treatment and care efforts must be accompanied by increased and integrated prevention efforts.

EFFECTIVE HIV PREVENTION MEASURES

Effective HIV prevention combines society-wide strategies with particular focus on those parts of the population most at risk. Whatever the extent of the spread of the epidemic young people-need to be at the centre of all HIV strategies--not least because most HIV infections occur during, or soon alter, adolescence. Strategies that work combine:

- AIDS life-skills education;
- mass media communication;
- access to condoms;
- voluntary counselling;
- testing and referral;
- treatment of sexually transmitted infections;
- involvement of parents and other adults; and
- efforts to improve young people's social and economic status.

In low-prevalence settings, a concentrated epidemic tends initially to be associated with certain high-risk contexts-- typically, sex work, injecting drug users and sex between men. Usually, these activities are also highly stigmatised. But the people at risk in these contexts are not isolated groups: they mix across populations, as confirmed by behavioural surveillance. However, early, large-scale interventions among these groups could stave off a potential epidemic. In high-prevalence settings, the epidemic is spread much more broadly throughout the general population. The higher the national HIV prevalence rate, the higher the proportion of people who must adopt safer behaviour if the epidemic is to be brought under control. Very high coverage with demonstrably effective interventions then becomes crucial. Whether in low- or high-prevalence areas the key to effective prevention is to apply essential prevention strategies to the realities of the epidemic, at the local, national or even regional levels. Twenty years into the HIV/AIDS epidemic, the majority of countries in the world still register national HIV prevalence rates of less than 1 per cent, for the global epidemic is still in its early stages. But two decades ago, there was no country in the world that had nationwide adult HIV prevalence rates above 1 per cent: today there are nearly 50 and, in 12 of them, national adult HIV prevalence is estimated to be more than 10 per cent.

HIV rates, reported as a national average, can be misleading. In populous countries, national adult HIV prevalence of, say. 2-3 per cent may nevertheless mean millions of infections. National HIV prevalence rates can also mask the concentrated nature of HIV epidemics in specific parts of the country and among specific populations. Large-scale epidemics always begin as localised outbreaks before spreading more widely across regions and communities.

In Nairobi, Kenya, HIV prevalence among female sex workers surged from 4 per cent in 1981 to 61 per cent in 1985, while prevalence among pregnant women rose from 0 per cent in 1981 to only 2 per cent in 1985, before its subsequent steep rise. The danger signs of impending epidemics are now familiar, but the exact pace of the epidemic's growth still cannot be predicted with certainty.

In Thailand, for example, the virus was first detected in 1984, but did not start spreading virulently among sex workers and their clients until five years later. Similarly, in the Nepalese city of Kathmandu, needle-sharing was rife in the early 1990s, yet HIV infections among injecting drug users stayed negligible for six or seven years before rising sharply to the point where, by 1997, nearly half the users were infected. In Indonesia, anonymous HIV testing of sex workers began in 1988 and, for almost a decade, registered virtually no HIV infection. The results were puzzling because other research was showing that sex work was common, condom use very low and other sexually transmitted infections highly prevalent.

The absence of a HIV epidemic may have been partly because sex workers in Indonesia had a relatively low turnover of partners--around seven in a week, on average, compared with over 30 a week in Thailand at the height of the HIV rise in that country. But new data suggest that there has been a surge in HIV infection among sex workers in some INDonesian locations.

Preventing Sexual Transmission of HIV

The World Health Organisation estimates that over 300 million people are infected each year with curable sexually transmitted infections, a large share of which occur among young people. The presence of such infections magnifies the risk of HIV transmission during unprotected sex as much as tenfold (since the infection creates additional entry points for the virus or facilitates viral replication). Many of these infections including the four most common: syphilis, gonorrhoea, *chlamydia* and trichomoniasis) can be cured relatively easily with antibiotic treatment. But lack of services, poor availability of drugs, limited access to diagnosis, and disparaging attitudes by service providers are barriers to more effective detection and treatment of sexually transmitted infections as part of HIV/AIDS prevention.

Safe sex is any sexual practice that reduces the risk of transmission of HIV from one person to another. The best protection is by sexual activities that prevent entry of infected semen, vaginal secretions or blood into the mouth, vagina or anus of the partner. These practices include:

(i) Staying in a mutually faithful relationship where both partners are uninfected.

(ii) Using a condom for all types of sexual intercourse (vaginal, anal or oral) to prevent body secretions containing HIV to come in contact with the skin or mucous membranes of the partner.

(iii) Avoiding penetrative sex and replacing it with masturbation, massage, dry kissing and hugging.

(iv) Avoiding sex when either partner has open sores or sexually transmitted diseases.

Usage of Condoms

Condoms are the most effective means of protection against the organisms that cause sexually transmitted infection, including HIV. They are effective only if they are used properly during every sexual intercourse. Without access to condoms, many other prevention strategies such as behavioural change communication and sexual and reproductive health education in schools, not to mention family planning campaigns lose much of their potential effectiveness.

The United Nations Population Fund estimates that the number of condoms needed to prevent HIV/ AIDS and other sexually transmitted infections will more than double in the next 15 years. Costs will rise from US $239 million in 2000 to an estimated US $557 million in 2015. This total does not include distribution, training or counselling costs. Low-income countries will need plans that address supply problems along with steady increases in donor support to meet condom costs.

Increasing condom accessibility and availability can increase condom use. In Brazil, there was *a* massive increase in the uptake of condoms when prices came down in the early 1990s. When Ford South Africa made mass condom distribution part of its HIV/AIDS strategy and put condom distribution machines in workplace toilets, uptake increased 25-fold. However, supply is not the only determinant of condom use. Almost everywhere, sexually active young people are denied information about condoms.

A recent analysis of study samples from eight countries in sub-Saharan Africa found that attitudes towards condom use also depended on the nature of relationships. In marital and regular relationships, many people said that they did not use condoms because they 'trusted their partner: in regular and casual relationships, people frequently cited a dislike or condoms. This suggests that condom promotion messages need to be tailored to context: couples in steady relationship may need to be convinced that using condoms is a primary means of caring for each other's health.

Condom programming works best as part of a comprehensive 'package' of interventions that include HIV/AIDS education, sexual health and human sexuality, and gender sensitivity training. Since it was first introduced by public health, authorities in Ratchaburi Province. Thailand's innovative 100 per cent Condom Use Programme for commercial sex has become known as one of the most effective HIV prevention measures ever.

Preventing HIV Transmission among Homosexuals

In varying degrees, male-to-male HIV transmission is a factor in all HIV epidemics. It has been the predominant mode of transmission of HIV in most high-income countries. In the USA, male-to-male sex accounted for the largest proportion (42 per cent) of annual new infections in 2000, while, in Australia, it accounted for 85 per cent of infections in 2000. Significant HIV prevalence among men who have sex with men has been detected in countries around the world. Where male-to-male sex is repressed legally or through strong social sanctions, men who have sex with men are at especially high risk of HIV infection, since they are harder to identify and reach with preventative services. Countering the discrimination and violence endured by men who have sex with men is therefore a vital part of an effective AIDS response.

Reliable data from countries as diverse as Brazil, Colombia, India, Mexico, Pakistan and Thailand confirm that many men who have unprotected sex with other men also have unprotected sex with women, in Latin America and the Caribbeans, the population of men who have sex with men is diverse, many of the men also have sex with women, HIV rates are significant and, as a result, the epidemic is steadily reaching their female partners. A recent study by the Senegalese National AIDS Commission in Dakar. Senegal, reported that 88 per cent of surveyed men who have sex with men also had sex with women, and 15 per cent were married. Only 14 per cent said they used condoms the last time they had sex. In addition. 37 per cent of the men surveyed reported that they had been raped in the previous year, some by policemen.

Gay communities in high-income countries have been at the forefront of the response to HIV/AIDS, and have mounted very successful prevention efforts, although a resurgence of unsafe sex among men who have sex with men shows the need to constantly renew and reinforce such efforts. In much of Africa and Asia, however, prevention efforts among men who have sex with men have barely begun.

In many middle-and low-income countries, male-to-male sex and HIV transmission tend to be statistically hidden and officially denied. In much of Africa, for example, male-to-male sex is scarcely acknowledged, although self-identified gay groups have been in existence for several years in South Africa and Zimbabwe. Similar groups have recently been formed in Kenya and Senegal.

The Bandhu Social Welfare Society (in Dhaka; Bangladesh); and Sahodaran (in Chennai, India) are community-based agencies providing both outreach and onsite services to men who have sex with men. 'Safe spaces in their central offices offer stigmatised and marginalised men an opportunity to socialise and to access a range of services. Bandhu Social Welfare Society has an innovative clinic service for sexually transmitted infection diagnosis and treatment and Sahodaran, has contributed strongly to national advocacy. Similarly, recent years have seen a series of prevention projects established in Eastern Europe and Central Asia by gay organisations in collaboration with local authorities, with support from UNAIDS Cosponsors and the UNAIDS Secretariat.

Preventing HIV Transmission among Sex Workers and Their Clients

Sex work is clandestine and illegal in most societies, which makes it difficult to gauge the numbers involved in it. But it is a global phenomenon and a powerful social and economic factors in many countries. By the International

Labour Organisation's estimates, the sex work industry accounted for more than 2 per cent of gross domestic product in four South-East Asian countries by the late 1990s. In countries where heterosexual intercourse is the main mode of HIV transmission. HIV/ epidemics tend to be concentrated initially aiming sex workers and their clients before becoming established in the wider population. A steep rise in HIV prevalence among sex workers is an alarm signal that HIV rates in the wider population are very likely to increase unless effective prevention efforts are introduced.

Where sex work is widespread but clandestine, this often reflects entrenched gender inequalities. In such places, men's social, economic and political status eclipses that of women, double standards encourage multiple partners for men but not for women, and women's limited educational and livelihood opportunities compel many into some form of sex work. While economic necessity is often the driving motivation for many in sex work, it is not necessarily the only one. Research in the Philippine sex industry, for instance, has found that some sex workers operating out of bars and clubs had worked in formal employment, but opted instead for the slightly lower earnings and risks of the sex trade over the long hours working on assembly lines. Others are coerced into sex work through violence, debt bondage, or trafficking.

It can be difficult or impossible for sex workers to insist on safe sex. Reluctant clients might react with violence or simply move on to someone willing to forego a condom. A recent analysis of condom use by sex workers in Kolkata. India, has found that clients were willing to pay almost double the fee for sex without, a condom.

Effective HIV prevention among sex workers addresses the social, economic and legal environments in which they live and work. Sex workers must be involved and empowered through the projects. Efforts must win the cooperation and support of control points in the sex industry, such as brothel owners, bar managers, pimps and the police. It is essential to tackle the prejudice that sex workers endure, and to weave other concerns into the programmes, such as care for their families and children.

When sex work is illegal, it is driven deeper underground, and prevention efforts become more difficult. Sex workers may be subject to police harassment, and carrying condoms can lead to arrest, fines or imprisonment. However, important victories have been won for the protection of sex workers' human rights. Sex workers involved in Bangladesh's Shakti project helped achieve an important court decision recognising sex work as a legal form of income-generation. In Papua New Guinea, the Transex project used a mixture of lobbying and activism to change the attitudes of the local police force, reducing its power over sex workers' lives and preventing it from obstructing the project.

Prevention of HIV Infection Via Blood Transfusion

The process of blood collection, transport, storage, testing and distribution, requires maintenance of a certain standard by application of effective quality control mechanism at all levels. Blood is a good medium for growth of any organism because of its nutrient value, adequate oxygen content and optimum temperature. Transfusion of infected blood, therefore, can lead to transmission of blood-borne diseases like hepatitis, syphilis, malaria, and HIV/AIDS. There is an overall acute shortage of blood. The gap between demand and supply of blood is continuously widening due to mushrooming of super-specialist hospitals in urban areas and continuous inappropriate use of blood. It has been estimated that approximately 30 per cent transfusions are either unnecessary or wasteful. Rational and appropriate use of blood and blood products and promotion of voluntary donation can help in overcoming this shortfall.

Blood transfusion should be given only when there is a definite indication to do so and its benefit outweighs the risk associated with it. It is necessary for appropriate use of simple alternatives to transfusion like crystalloids or colloids that are safer and more cost effective. If transfusion cannot be avoided then specific blood component should be used if possible. Reducing the exposure of patient TO different donors will also decrease the risk of transfusion-transmitted diseases. This is of importance in a paediatric patient requiring small quantity of blood every day or on alternate days, who may be transfused with small quantities of blood separated from a single blood unit.

All injections should be avoided as far as possible. Oral medications should be used instead. If injections cannot be avoided, make sure that the needles and syringes are either new disposable ones or appropriately sterilised. Avoid all addictive drugs. If not possible, it is better to use them orally. If injecting drugs cannot be avoided, then the injecting equipment should not be shared. If not possible to avoid sharing equipment, then either boil the equipment for 20 minutes or use fresh bleach solution.

Prevention of HIV Infection among Injecting Drug Users

The illicit drug trade has, over the past 25 years, grown into a multi-billion-dollar industry that spans the planet. By the end of 1999, injecting drug use was being reported in 136 countries: in 114 of them, HIV cases resulting from injecting drug use had been reported. Drug trafficking is now a global phenomenon, touching some 170 countries and territories. It is estimated that up to 10 million people worldwide inject drugs.

Asia is estimated to have the largest number of injecting-drug-related HIV cases. Injecting drug use is also a major factor in HIV epidemics in North America. Western Europe and in parts of Latin America, the Middle East and North Africa. In some Eastern European countries, especially in countries of the former Soviet Union, injecting drug use is driving major HIV/ AIDS epidemics among young people, and many outreach programmes report rising numbers of sexually active teenage drug users.

Injecting-drug-related HIV epidemics do not remain limited to injecting drug users. Most injecting drug users are young, male and sexually active. They are likely to acquire or transmit the HIV virus not only by sharing injecting equipment but also through sexual intercourse with regular or casual partners. Injecting drug use also overlaps profoundly with the sex trade, with users often buying sex, or selling sex to finance their drug dependencies. In 2000, in Hanoi. Vietnam. 20 per cent of street-based female sex workers reported recent drug injection, while 23 per cent of male injecting drug users bought sex; in Bangladesh, the corresponding figures were 14 per cent and 50-75 per cent respectively.

Stopping the spread of HIV among injecting drug users requires a comprehensive approach, including drug-dependency treatment and rehabilitation; HIV/AIDS education: access to clean needles/syringes and condoms; legal and social services; and voluntary HIV testing and counselling and psychosocial support. It also requires efforts to deter people (especially young people) from initiating injecting drug use. There is strong evidence to show that effective and humane drug treatment not only reduces drug abuse, but also diminishes HIV risk. A basic ethical principle is that drug control policies must reduce, not augment, the HIV risk faced by drug users, and HIV prevention activities must not inadvertently promote drug abuse.

Small, isolated prevention efforts might slow the pace of the epidemic, but not for long, as Nepal's experience has shown Needle exchange programmes there began as early as 1991: by 1995, some researchers were claiming that the interventions had averted a HIV epidemic among injecting drug users. But, by 1997, almost half the users tested in Kathmandu were infected with HIV. The needle-exchange programme was too limited and too localised to have a powerful, lasting impact. It had to be expanded. Needle and syringe programmes have also been expanded elsewhere, notably in some countries in Europe and in Australia. In 2000, in England and Wales, there were 420 syringe-distribution programmes, distribute 27 million syringes, equivalent to 180-540 syringes per injecting drug user per year.

Evidence from high- and low-income countries shows that effective prevention and care programmes can be mounted despite the marginalisation, social stigma and legally penalising environment that mark injecting drug users' lives. But the programmes tend to be most successful when laws and police practices facilitate outreach work and service provision to injecting drug users.

For many years, Manipur in India was emblematic of a region in the grip of a rising injecting drug-related HIV epidemic. By the late 1990s, there were already an estimated 40.000 injecting drug users in Manipur, as many as 60 per cent of whom were HIV-positive. To many observers, it seemed a lost cause. But, after studies had revealed that most of the users shared injecting equipment because they feared arrest if caught with needles and syringes, the Society for HIV/AIDS and Lifelines Operations (SHALOM) took the bold step of setting up a needle and syringe-exchange programme in Churachandpur township. Police were consulted and persuaded not to harass Shalom workers or users found with injecting equipment. HIV incidence among users dropped from almost 77 per cent in 1997 to just under 59 per cent in 2001--still high, but a marked decrease. Persuaded by the effectiveness of the programme, the Manipur Minister of State for Health integrated the approach into the official State AIDS policy.

Bigger official obstacles were cleared in Ukraine, where, in 1998, the parliament added to a HIV/AIDS law the State's guarantee that it would work to facilitate the provision of needle-exchange services for injecting drug users. This hard-won law reform also abolished the mandatory testing of users. Political and public opinion at first had been fearful that the changes would spur drug use and other social problems. But a strong information campaign and widespread public debate gradually convinced voters and legislators that the reforms were ultimately going to benefit all society. Currently, in 2002, 37 needle-exchange projects operate in the country, and are estimated to reach around 20 per cent of all users.

In Brazil, a law was approved by Congress in 2002, authorising the Ministry of Health to establish national policies for specific HIV programmes targeting injecting drug users. A national survey among injecting drug users showed that consistent use of condoms in this population increased from 42 per cent in 1999 to 65 per cent in the year 2000. In the same period, syringe- and needle-sharing decreased from 70 per cent to 41 per cent. As a result, between 1996 and 2000, HIV prevalence among injecting drug users dropped in several cities. In Santos, Sao Paulo State, the drop was from 65 per cent to 42 per cent; in Salvador, from 49 per cent to 7 per cent; and in the city of Rio de Janeiro, from 25 per cent to 8 per cent.

Drug substitution programmes, along with a range of other health and referral services, have been successfully introduced in some places. An example is the Mexican non-governmental organisation, Companeros AC, which has run a programme since the mid-1990s, promoting detoxification and rehabilitation alongside specific HIV-prevention efforts targeting injecting drug users. It helps injecting drug users make behavioural changes that are realistic for them and that are most likely to be sustained--from outright cessation of drug use to adopting less harmful habits.

Fieldwork is carried out in prisons as well as in the wider community. Information leaflets are distributed, along with packages containing condoms, bleach, and education leaflets. Rehabilitation services incorporate complementary treatments such as acupuncture and herbal medicine. Education and support are provided to the families and partners of people who inject drugs.

Prevention of HIV/AIDS from Mother to Child

Prevention of vertical transmission of HIV from mother to child is possible in the following ways:

(i) Intrapartum

(a) Delivery in hospital.

(b) Antiretroviral therapy--AZT or Nevirapine.

(c) Do not do amniotomy, foetal scalp blood sampling.

foetal scalp electrode monitoring or umbilical blood sampling.

(d) Role of Caesarian Section.

(ii) Antepartum

(a) Counselling in the antenatal period and HIV testing.

(b) Choice of MTP or continuation of pregnancy.

(c) Correct diet and treatment of anaemia.

(d) Discontinue smoking and illicit drugs.

(e) Regular check up.

(f) Treat RTI/STI.

(g) Detect and treat opportunistic infections.

(h) Antiretroviral therapy.

(iii) Postpartum

(a) Immediate bath to baby.

(b) Breast-feeding vs safer alternatives.

(c) Anti-retroviral therapy to the baby.

HIV infected individuals may suffer from a variety of disorders and develop signs which are suggestive of being infected by HIV/AIDS. Since sophisticated blood tests may not be available in many developing countries. WHO has laid down clinical criteria for the provisional diagnosis of AIDS. The presence of at least two major signs and one minor sign can be an indication for AIDS provided other causes of depleted immunity are ruled out.

Major Signs

(i) Weight loss >10 per cent of body weight.

(ii) Fever for more than one month, intermittent or continuous.

(iii) Chronic diarrhoea for more than one month.

Minor Signs

(i) Persistent cough for more than one month,

(ii) Generalised dermatitis,

(iii) Recurrent herpes zoster,

(iv) Oro-pharyngeal candidiasis,

(v) Chronic progressive and disseminated herpes simplex infection,

(vi) Generalised lymphadenopathy.

Counselling and Testing

Counselling and testing has been shown to have a role in both HIV prevention and as an entry point to care. It provides people with an opportunity to learn and accept their HIV status in a confidential environment. This become an integral part of HIV prevention programmes in many countries as it a relatively cost effective intervention in preventing HIV transmission. In India, as HIV testing becomes simpler to perform with the advent of newer kits, the National AIDS Control Organisation has plans for the expansion of testing facilities to all corners of the country in a phased manner.

HIV testing services should be designated to address the multiple needs and rights of individuals at risk or already infected. Such efforts to reduce stigma and discrimination seek to 'normalise' community perceptions of HIV infection and AIDS, and make counselling services available to all who seek them, regardless of their willingness to he tested.

The diagnosis of HIV testing has traditionally been made by detecting antibodies against HIV. There has been rapid evolution in diagnostic technology since the first HIV antibody tests became commercially available. Besides

ELISA, newer rapid and simple tests are available which are comparable to ELISA on sensitivity and specificity. In addition they are easy to perform in limited resource settings like district hospitals and more cost-effective than ELISA. The success of counselling and testing strategy largely depends on the availability of cheap testing facilities that give results in the shortest possible time. This makes the rapid tests an attractive option where the client can be subjected to a pretest counselling, test result and post-test counselling in one session.

Counselling should be offered before taking an HIV test. In this process the counselor prepares the client for the test by explaining what an HIV test is and also by correcting myths and misinformation about HIV/AIDS. This counselling can also be provided to groups to reduce costs and can be backed up by providing printed information. Post-test counselling should always be offered. The idea is to help clients to understand their test results and initiate adaptation to their sero-positive or sero-negative status. When the test is sero-positive, the counsellor tells the client the result clearly and sensitively, providing emotional support and discussing how he/she will cope.

The counsellor must ensure that the person has immediate emotional support from a partner, relative or friend. Sharing one's HIV status with a sexual partner is important to enable the use of safer sexual practices and should be encouraged. Counselling is also important when the test result is negative. While the client is likely to feel relief, the counsellor needs to discuss changes in behaviour that can help the client to stay negative.

HIV/AIDS is a disease with long incubation period. People suffering from this condition require long-term, continuous treatment. Hospital care in such conditions is not feasible. So, home-based care is absolutely necessary for such cases. Home-based care has some specific objectives:

(i) Formation of indispensable teams, which will train the family members who will provide social support and teach prevention. They will develop referral network linking health services with NGOs.

(ii) *Clinical management:* A proper diagnosis and treatment.

About two decades have passed since HIV/AIDS has entered the medical horizon. As yet, no curative treatment has been found. However, four years after the virus was discovered, the first drug for treatment of HIV infection was discovered. Scientists discovered agents that act on the life cycle of the virus in the body and stop viral replication.

The first drug, which was discovered in 1987, acted on the reverse transcriptase enzyme to prevent formation of pro- virus DNA. Since then, various drugs acting on reverse transcriptase have been discovered. Two groups of drugs:

(i) Nucleoside Analogues and

(ii) Non-nucleoside analogues were discovered till 1998.

In 1998, another group of drugs called protease inhibitors was discovered and announced in the World Congress of AIDS in Vancouver. These were the drugs, which acted on the enzyme protease, which helped in the maturation of m-RNA to mature, virions. All these anti retroviral drugs act on various stages of the life cycle of the virus in the human body and stop the replication of the virus but do not eradicate the virus out of the human cell where they are firmly integrated.

Recent Developments

Potential technologies currently being pursued also hold the promise of radically changing the landscape of HIV/AIDS prevention. The most prominent are microbicides and vaccines against HIV.

Microbicides

As a form of 'chemical condom' that can be self-administered microbicides could increase the options for women and men who find it difficult or impossible to persuade their partners to use a condom. Acceptability studies in South Africa, Uganda and Zimbabwe suggest that women who seldom or never use condoms could reduce their overall risk of infection if an effective microbicide were available to them at low cost.

Applied inside the vagina or rectum, a microbicide is intended to prevent infection with HIV and possibly, other bacterial and viral sexually transmitted infections, it can be produced as a gel, cream, suppository, sponge or in other forms, and may also have contraceptive (spermicidal) prcperties. The ideal product would be odourless and colourless, and therefore undetectable to partners who refuse ether forms of protection.

After the disappointment of the Phase III trial of nonoxynol-9 gel, an estimated 56 new products are in various stages of development, from pre-clinical stages to Phase III effectiveness trials. While no major pharmaceutical company has thus far invested in the development of a microbicide, research into this preventive option has recently been spurred by several grants from the Bill and Melinda Gates Foundation. The International Working Group on Microbicides, which includes public agencies from around the world among its members, continues to promote and facilitate the development of microbicides.

Vaccines

Research to find a vaccine against HIV has been making steady progress in the past 10 years. Unfortunately, 'steady' is not fast enough for all the people who could benefit from it. Even if current attempts to speed up the research process and programmes for the introduction of vaccines are successful, there is little chance that vaccination against HIV will be available on a large scale before the end of the decade.

An estimated US $400--500 million is currently spent on HIV vaccine research annually, with most of this going into basic research. Institutions involved in the global HIV vaccine effort include the US National Institutes of Health, the International AIDS Vaccine Initiative (IAVI), the US Centers for Disease Control and Prevention, the French *Agence Nationale de Recherches sur le SIDA* (ANRS), the European Community (through the EUROVAC programme), and several biotechnology and pharmaceutical companies. National AIDS vaccine research programmes are ongoing in Australia, Canada, Japan, Sweden, the United Kingdom and the United States of America. Low- and middle-income countries (including Brazil, China, Cuba. Haiti, India. Kenya, South Africa. Thailand, Trinidad and Tobago, and Uganda) are also actively involved in vaccine development and trials. WHO and UNAIDS have been actively supporting these national AIDS vaccine programmes.

Despite all this activity, the peculiarities of the HIV virus make finding a vaccine difficult and expensive. HIV differs from most other infectious diseases in that the virus directly attacks white blood cells that are central to directing the body's immune responses, leaving them incapable of controlling infection or preventing disease.

'Classical' vaccines, based on an entire microorganism (viruses or bacteria) that has been killed or rendered harmless, may not be safe enough to use against HIV as they could lead to HIV infection.

Experimental HIV vaccines are therefore primarily based on parts of the virus, which makes the development of a vaccine even more challenging. The multiple variants of HIV pose a further complication. Ten subtypes of the HIV-1 virus have been identified, and are distributed in different parts of the world. Researchers do not yet know whether a broadly protective vaccine will be possible or if a separate vaccine will be needed for each subtype.

The most prevalent HIV subtypes are A and C, present in different regions in Africa, but the majority of the vaccines currently in trials are modelled on the genetic profile of subtype B--the one predominant in high-income countries. Finally, HIV vaccine research remains a 'highrisk/ low-return investment for private sector industry. This is only partly because the greatest need for the vaccine is among low-income countries. An even greater obstacle--at least currently--is the inadequate scientific understanding of the mechanisms by which the virus evades the body's natural immune responses. Consequently, it is not known exactly what immune responses are necessary to prevent or control HIV infection.

Developing a HIV vaccine is an arduous process. Experimental vaccines are first tested on animals, and the best vaccine candidates are then selected for possible testing on humans. Testing is then carried out on healthy volunteers in three phases.

Phase I trials are done on 20-40 volunteers to confirm the vaccine's safety and whether it triggers useful HIV-specific immune responses.

Phase II tests involve hundreds of volunteers to further check safety and assess the potency of immune responses.

Phase III tests can last up to four years and involve field trials with thousands of volunteers, some of whom receive the vaccine while others form a control group.

Extremely complicated from the logistical, scientific and ethical points of view, these trials assess whether the candidate vaccine protects against HIV infection or the onset of AIDS. Definitive results of the first Phase III trials of a candidate vaccine based on gp 120 (an external protein of HIV) are expected in 2003.

The first Phase III trial, with 5400 volunteers, has been ongoing in the United States. Canada and the Netherlands since 1998, and is based on subtype B. The second Phase III trial began in 1999 in Thailand, and is based on the B and E subtypes prevalent there, involving 2500 volunteers. Planning is under way to initiate a Phase III trial of another approach in Thailand in 2003, and additional candidate vaccines are entering Phase I/II trials.

An African AIDS Vaccine Programme, announced in Nairobi in June 2000, is bringing together African scientists, governments and institutions. They aim to complete at least one efficacy trial by 2007.

While a useable vaccine is still many years away, discussion has begun on how to implement vaccination programmes once one exists. Usually, vaccines only arrive in low-and middle-income countries many years after they have recouped their costs in high-income countries. This cannot be allowed to occur with effective HIV vaccines, which need to be rapidly available, and affordable to all who need them.

Mechanisms to ensure simultaneous access to AIDS vaccines in both low- and high-income countries must be prepared long before a vaccine is developed, in order to provide quick access to those who need it. The International AIDS Vaccine Initiative and others are proposing significant changes to existing approaches to vaccine production, licensing, pricing, purchasing and distribution. Among other issues is the need to harmonise national regulations and international guidelines governing vaccine approval and use.

An important technical challenge will be that of creating the necessary production capacity, and supporting it with reliable estimates of demand for specific vaccines. Many of the challenges in ensuring that a vaccine is available--and affordable--are similar to those relating to expanding access to antiretroviral drugs.

Differential pricing, together with financial support from donors, will almost certainly be necessary for low-income countries. Technical assistance and coordination by international agencies will be needed. There are policy conundrums, too. Since the vaccination will not immediately be available to everyone, costs and benefits have to be calculated to determine where the initial focus should be Policymakers must also decide what to do if the first available vaccines are only marginally effective or have significant side effects.

WHO. UNAIDS and IAVI have collaborated on a study aimed at estimating the need for, and probable uptake of, preventative vaccines based on two potential scenarious a low moderate-efficacy vaccine (30-50 per cent effective) and a high-efficacy vaccine (80-90 per cent effective). A vaccination programme using a low/ moderate-efficacy vaccine would need to be accompanied by intensive positive-behaviour counselling, so as not to undermine existing prevention efforts. Furthermore, it would be likely to have the most benefit if vaccination were targeted at populations most vulnerable to HIV infection. A high-efficacy vaccine could be delivered to larger segments of the general population. Although it is difficult to predict the uptake of vaccines, in the absence of information on the cost of the vaccine itself and on the requirements for delivery, the study concluded that the probable uptake would be far less than the estimated need, both for a low/moderate- and a high-efficacy vaccine.

The unique stigma associated with HIV/AIDS may significantly hinder the uptake of HIV vaccination, once it becomes available. Discrimination faced by many of the communities most vulnerable to HIV infection may prevent individuals from coming forward for vaccination, particularly if programmes are focused only at individuals who might be at high risk of infection. When an effective HIV vaccine is available, the international community and affected countries will have to make many critical decisions on how to use it. Extra investment in HIV/AIDS prevention and control will be necessary.

REFERENCES

Alexander P.. "Contextual risk versus behaviour: The impact of the legal, social and economic context of sex work on individual risk taking", 2001.

Burrows d. Landman W. "Harm reduction: A key component of fighting AIDS in Russia". *Sexual Health Exchange* 2001-2: p. 5-7, 2002.

Centers for Disease Control and Prevention. Need *for Sustained HIV* Prevention for Gay and Bisexual *Men: HIV Infections Continue at High Levels among Men of All Races with Dramatic Impact among Men of Color.* Atlanta: National Center for HIV, STD and TB Prevention. 2000.

Crofts N., et al. "Harm Reduction in Asia: A successful response to hidden epidemics", *AIDS:* 12 (supplement B): S109-S115. 1998.

Delor F. Hubert M.. "Revisiting the concept of 'vulnerability'". *Social Science & Medicine:* 50: 1557-1570. 2000.

Eastwood. A., and A. Maynard. 1988. Treating AIDS Patients: Is it Ethical to be Efficient" Paper presented at the First International Conference on the Global Impact of AIDS. London. March.

Egal F. Valstar A., *HIV/AIDS and nutrition: helping families and communities to cope,* Rome: Food and Agriculture Organisation, 2000.

Engender Health, *STI-HIV-Prevention—Quick Reference Cards for Health Care Provides-What Every Client Should Know,* New York, 2001.

Grosskurth H et al.. "Control of sexually transmitted diseases for HIV prevention: understanding the implications of the Mwanza and Rakai trials". *The Lancet.* 2000.

Institute of Medicine, National Academy of Sciences. *Mobilising Against AIDS*, Cambridge, Mass, Harvard University Press, 1986.

South African AIDS Training (SAT) Programme. *Counselling Guidelines on Survival Skills for People Living with HIV, 2001.*

UNAIDS. "Innovative approaches to HIV prevention". *Best Practice Collection,* Geneva, 2000.

UNAIDS. Report on the global HIV/AIDS Epidemic, 2002.

UNDP. "HIV/AIDS: *Implication, for Poverty Reduction.*" New York, 2001.

World Bank, *Confronting AIDS: public priorities in a global epidemic,* Oxford: Oxford University Press for the World Bank. 1999.

CHAPTER 4

Effective Counselling: Methods & Techniques

It must be kept in mind that Counselling is different from providing a medical service where providers generally give treatment, health information, advice and instructions to service users. This partnership model means that attitudes are very important in counselling. The counsellor's attitudes as a counsellor are very important. Sexuality, is a sensitive subject and unless the counsellor show the clients that she/he care about and respect them, they will not be able to talk openly about their lives and feelings.

Effective counselling is important in helping people with concerns about sexuality, STI and HIV. Many people feel unable to talk about them because of embarrassment or fear of rejection. If they do, they may not receive the emotional support, information and skills they require. Fears about the future, guilt, anger and despair may overwhelm them. They may not feel able to talk to their partner about sexual problems. safer sex or an STI/HIV diagnosis. These situations are complex and clients need time to talk them over and make good decisions.

Counselling empowers individuals to prevent transmission of HIV by enabling them to cope with the personal implications of an HIV diagnosis and to make informed personal decisions, including those related to sexuality and reproduction. Counsellors can help the affected persons adopt new lifestyles, and assist them to retain their identities, independence, privacy, social status and self-worth. This can then reduce the risk of negative outcomes, re-infection, and transmission of infection to others.

Models

There are several models of counselling where the counsellor can use his skills. GATHER is one that is often used in contraceptive counselling.

Greet the clients
Ask the clients why they have come and about their situations
Tell the clients how you can help them
Help the clients to make their own decisions
Explain how to use the methods they have chosen
Return visits are arranged to see how they are getting on.

This model was designed for contraceptive counselling, but counsellor can adapt it for STI/HIV.

REDA is another model, which is more open and flexible
Rapport is developed between counsellor and client
Explore the problem, situation and options for change
Decide on the best option
Act on the decision.

Role of Counselling

Counsellors have many opportunities to counsel clients on other sexual and reproductive health issues, including STI/HIV because:

- Counsellors see people who are in sexual relationships and may be at risk of STI/HIV.
- Counsellors distribute male and female condoms, the only methods that protect, against STI/HIV.
- Clients need protection from unwanted pregnancy and STI/HIV.
- Clients need to take risk of STI/HIV into account when they make a decision about which contraceptive to use.
- Some counsellors are used to talking about sexual issues.
- Counsellors may talk about gender relations, which affect risk of STI/HIV.
- Counsellors can discuss concerns about STI, including signs and symptoms and refer.
- Counsellors can be aware of the possibility of sexual abuse and support clients.

Some providers worry that integrating STI/HIV into their family planning programme will have a negative impact on their services. In fact it may improve quality for the following reasons:

- The client is looked at in a holistic way, which helps the client with family planning and sexual life generally. Clients feel that the counsellor cares about them as people rather than contraceptive acceptors.

- The use of existing facilities is maximised because counsellors are already trained, experienced and trusted.
- The counsellor can reach a wider group of clients with unmet needs, including young people, men and those not at risk of pregnancy.
- Having a package of different health services helps to prevent stigma.
- The services may have more access to government and other support services, including traditional healers.

There are some differences between counselling on family planning and counselling on STI/HIV, which the counsellor need to address in his plan to integrate services. It is important to use a participatory process in which leaders, managers and staff at all levels explore the costs and benefits of integrating different types of sexual health services into the existing programmes. The counsellor then has to make a joint decision on which services, if any to offer in relation to local needs and service gaps and values, identity and resources.

The counsellor may feel that STI/HIV counselling is an additional task that reveals problems that are difficult to resolve. He/she need to take part in the decision to integrate STI/HIV counselling, given a chance to express his/her fears and to identify the support needs. People may see family 3 planning clinics as places where 'respectable' married women go for contraception, to do with fertility, not talking about a potentially fatal disease passed through sex. The counsellor may fear that the change of image will drive away clients.

Counsellors need knowledge of the medical and a social issues of HIV and contacts with the family and community to address them. There is more stigma, judgmental attitudes and secrecy around STI/HIV than family planning. This makes it harder to talk about openly and the consequences of disclosure more difficult. Counsellors have limited ways to help clients with these issues. It is important to work for changes in attitudes towards STI/HIV, perhaps by collaborating with other organisations.

The counsellor need knowledge of available resources for STI/HIV prevention, support and care in the locality. Offer all existing clients the opportunity for STI/HIV prevention counselling. The counsellor might make the services more accessible to groups who are also vulnerable to STI/HIV, such as young people, men or single women. He/she may need to change his/her image and to attract these groups and provide them with confidential, acceptable services. If couples agree, it can be helpful to counsel them together. This can build trust, help them to communicate more easily and make joint decisions about HIV testing and safer sex options.

People who are motivated to counsel are more likely to make good, empathetic counsellors. Managers should only give counselling duties to providers who feel committed to it. The counsellor need to:

- Train existing service providers.
- Re-organise clinics to make better use of staff time.
- Recruit new staff and/or volunteers.

Lay volunteers are often trained in HIV counselling to fill the gaps in provision. The counsellor need to:

- Integrate the work of volunteers into that of other health workers.
- Consult them about ways to maintain their motivation.
- Give agreed rewards for the time and energy that they devote to a difficult task. In poor communities this should usually include material rewards.
- Design training courses that are tailored to meet the specific needs of the volunteers.
- Give frequent refresher training to update knowledge and skills.
- Provide practical items for example, notebooks, condoms, penis models, and leaflets.
- Respect and value the work of the volunteers and acknowledge their generosity to others.
- Arrange frequent meetings with volunteers to share achievements and problems, build support.

Counsellors need adequate training on all aspects of sexuality and STI/HIV counselling and supervised practice and support. They may not have covered sexuality, STI/HIV and gender relations adequately in previous training or may not have applied the training. Helping people to adopt safer sex practices ay be more difficult than helping them to use contraception if it involves both partners in lifestyle changes and requires discussing intimate sexual practices. The counsellor need to spend time on relationship issues and enhancing clients assertiveness and communication skills.

Topics need to cover basic information about STIs and HIV/AIDS, transmission routes, risk factors, possible and available interventions, pre-and post-HIV antibody test counselling and prevention counselling.

Counsellors may need new knowledge and skills, for example, on interventions to reduce HIV transmission from pregnant women to children. Health care workers may have had little training in HIV/AIDS care and may have similar: attitudes to community members. Some issues, such as the benefits of replacement feeding, will contradict previous advice. Counsellors will need time and help to explore their own attitudes to sexual issues and how these may affect their counseling. This presents new challenges in being tolerant and talking about perhaps disapproved sexual practices.

Managers must acknowledge the importance of counselling on STI/HIV for their organisations, appreciate the staff who do this and allow them sufficient time to counsel. Many counsellors experience stress as a result of counselling on, HIV. Managers need to provide regular support to minimise "burn out" and avoid losing valuable staff, Counsellors need to regularly change their tasks and have breaks from HIV counselling and also have access to counselling themselves.

Discussing HIV may raise personal anxieties for providers and may affect their ability to counsel others. Confidential counselling support and testing should be available. Language barriers may be a problem which confidential lay interpreters can help with. Knowledge of HIV/AIDS is changing fast Counsellors need to keep uptodate to provide accurate information to clients, for example by updates from local HIV experts and the internet.

The counsellor need to change the organisation of his/her clinic to enhance privacy and client flows to enable young people and men to access the services. Some clinics have little time for counselling each client. There are a number of solutions to this problem:

(i) *Move out of the clinic:* The clinic may not be the best place to counsel, particularly for clients for whom sexual activity is not approved. Community-based counsellors can meet people privately in a suitable place and provide more-relaxed and accessible counselling.

(ii) *Group information-giving:* Group information-giving can help to provide more people with knowledge but counsellors still need to check that clients understand the facts in relation to their own lives. Between 10 and 20 people in a group gives opportunities for discussion. The counsellor need to:

(a) Warn the group that you cannot guarantee confidentiality and it is safest to talk about issues in a general way rather than disclose personal information. This can happen later in the individual counselling sessions.

(b) Give the basic facts about HIV/AIDS. transmission routes, what the test can tell you potential advantages and disadvantages of having the test and the process of counselling and testing. Give the information in a clear and interesting way that relates to people's lives.

(c) Ask the group if they have any questions and encourage discussion through the information giving.

(iii) *Group counselling:* A group of about ten people who feel comfortable to talk together can discuss thing in more-depth. For example, single sex groups of a similar age and status, couples or families.

(a) Explain that people may wish to share their feelings and experiences but they must understand that confidentiality *is* not guaranteed in a group.

(b) Build rapport, explore issues around testing, options for risk reduction and coping mechanisms.

(c) Encourage sharing of successful strategies for safer sex and coping and help people to gain more understanding of their options, the test and their own feelings.

(iv) *HIV antibody counselling in antenatal clinics:* In some countries, HIV testing of all pregnant women is compulsory. All HIV testing should be voluntary, with women making an informed decision whether to be tested or not after counselling. Women attend antenatal clinics for the purpose of their own health and the health of their child. They are unprepared for HIV testing and often find it traumatic. They often have no signs or symptoms of STI or HIV and little knowledge about it. Women usually attend the antenatal clinic alone and this can make it very difficult to tell their partner about the test result, Providers and clients at the antenatal clinic may not be sufficiently aware of the level of confidentiality required in HIV testing. There is little privacy in many antenatal clinics. Therefore:

(a) Counsel in privacy so that women feel comfortable to discuss sexual risk factors.

(b) Provide a space where accompanying children can play with supervision.

(c) Share confidential information about clients with providers to ensure that pregnant women get treatment and support and to reassure providers that they are not being put at risk.

(d) HIV test counselling and ongoing support takes-longer than the usual antenatal interview.

(e) Giving pre-test information in groups can save time during counselling.

Ideally counsellors should provide services at times convenient to their clients. This may be easier if they are working outside the clinic, in the community. Counsellors need time to do good counselling on STI/HIV. Pre-HIV test counselling takes at less 30 minutes and post-test counselling after a positive result may take more than an hour and need to continue. Managers must recognise the time needed and plan accordingly.

Consider human, material and financial resources carefully and realistically before making decisions about what type of counselling to offer. Family planning and other local services may not have resources such as drugs needed to help clients who test HIV positive or have a STI. The counsellor need to tailor counselling to available resources, seek funding before starting or form partnerships with other organisations.

Counselling Among Partners

Partner counselling/notification involves the process of contacting sexual and/or injecting partners of an HIV-positive person in order to advise these partners that they may have been exposed to HIV and to encourage them to attend for HIV counselling, testing and, where applicable, treatment. The objectives of this kind of disclosure are to prevent HIV transmission to people who may be exposed either sexually or through needle-sharing and to improve care and support for people living with HIV or AIDS.

Partner counselling can be undertaken by the source client or patient him/herself, by the health rare provider or through the combined efforts of both.

(i) *Source referral:* HIV-positive people are encouraged to counsel partners concerning their possible exposure to HIV. This takes place without the direct involvement of health care providers. In this approach, the health rare provider works with the HIV-positive person regarding the nature of the information to be passed on to their partner(s) and ways of doing it.

(ii) *Provider referral:* An HIV-positive person gives the name(s) of his/her partner(s) to a health care provider who then confidentially counsels the partner(s) directly. In this approach, the health care provider does not disclose the name of the HIV-positive person to the partner, but only provides the information that the partner is likely to have been exposed to HIV infection. This is done with the consent of the source client or patient.

(iii) *Conditional referral:* The health care provider of the source client or patient obtains the names of his/her sexual/drug-injecting partner(s), but allows the source client a period of time to counsel the partner(s) him/ herself. If partners are not counselled within this time period, the health care provider counsels the partners without naming the source patient or client concerned.

Partner counselling/notification has a long history as one possible aspect of the public health response to STIs other than HIV. such as syphilis and gonorrhoea. There is current debate whether, in the context of the transmission of HIV, the status and/or name of an HIV-positive person should be disclosed mandatorily to his or her sexual or drug-injecting partners. This is a particular concern in Africa and Asia where many women are being infected by their husbands or regular partners who do not reveal their HIV status or practise safe sex.

In the history of partner counselling, there are no clear data indicating that the mandatory counselling of partners is more effective in preventing transmission than the voluntary counselling of partners. It does appear that when people think that they will be forced to notify their partners, or that their status will be revealed without their consent, they choose not to attend for STI testing, counselling or other prevention and care services. This has been true in the case of syphilis and gonorrhoea even though, unlike HIV, these are curable and attract much less stigma and discrimination than HIV/AIDS.

It is even more likely that a policy of mandatory partner counselling will deter people from using HIV testing and counselling services, because there is greater incentive to fear testing and disclosure because of the serious stigma and discrimination surrounding HIV/AIDS. In fact, the reality is that, in many hospitals and clinics in low-income countries, disclosure of HIV status to sexual partners and others, such as family members, often takes place without consent. This happens because there are insufficient resources and personnel to store information in a way that respects privacy and/or because health care providers do not understand the professional duties of confidentiality and informed consent and their importance in the management of HIV/AIDS. This failure of health authorities to protect the privacy and autonomy of patients deters many people in these countries from seeking HIV counselling, testing and care.

It is not possible or practical to implement a large-scale scheme of mandatory partner counselling. It is virtually impossible to force people to test mandatorily for HIV. to retest periodically and to continue to inform partners, as would be necessary. Nor do people always know, or remember, the names of their sexual partners. Nor is it possible to force them to reveal them. Finally, it is very costly to train and employ staff to trace and counsel all those whose names are given.

However, it appears that mandatory partner counselling schemes are not necessary because voluntary partner counselling schemes can accomplish the critical goals. Voluntary partner counselling schemes can help to create a climate of confidence which will attract people to HIV, testing and counselling services so that more people learn of their HIV status. Among those who do attend health care facilities and are faced with a decision whether to notify partners or not, it appears that most, people agree to do so on a voluntary basis, after counselling. In the context of a generally voluntary partner counselling programme, the small number of cases where persons refuse to notify their partners can be taken care of on an individual basis. Thus, for reasons of principle and because it is more feasible and capable of success, ethical partner counselling is encouraged by UNAIDS and WHO.

Ethical partner counselling is based on the informed consent of the source client or patient and, where possible, maintains the confidentiality of the source client or patient: the is, his/her name is not revealed to the partners being counselled. This will often be extremely difficult to maintain in the context of marital relationships, and requires the provision of counselling and support to both spouses to ensure the prospect of abuse and discrimination is minimised or eliminated.

Ethical partner counselling also takes into account the serious consequence of not counselling partners--possible HIV infection. This consequence requires an ethical weighing of the benefits and harm that are likely to occur if and when there is refusal on the part of an HIV-positive person to counsel partners.

UNAIDS and WHO encourage ethical partner counselling programmes which:

- employ serious counselling and persuasion toward counselling of partners;
- empower the health care provider, when the source client refuses to notify his/her partner, to make ethical decision based on the potential harm and benefits to the parties and decide whether to counsel the partner(s) without the consent of the source client:
- provide social and legal support for the source client and other relevant parties (spouses, partners, family members to protect them from physical abuse, discrimination and stigma which may result from partner counselling.

UNAIDS and WHO advocate that there be greater

exploration of concepts and practices concerning partner counselling which are culturally appropriate, ethically sound and effective in achieving prevention and care goals. One example is the concept of "shared confidentiality". The aim of shared confidentiality is to promote better support, care and prevention for individuals, families and communities affected by HIV/ AIDS.

In communities where shared confidentiality has been a practice of community-based organisations, there has been an increase in community discussion of HIV/AIDS and a decrease in the stigma and discrimination surrounding HIV/AIDS. It has therefore helped to open up the HIV/ AIDS epidemic in positive and supportive ways.

In Uganda and some other African countries, this notion of shared confidentiality has been developed by communities. NGOs and health care providers. A person affected by HIV is encouraged, and voluntarily chooses, to disclose his status to a range of people from whom he can get support.

There will be some cases where an HIV-positive person (source client) does not wish to, and may refuse to, notify his her partner(s) or allow them to be counselled by the health care provider. Such refusal is most often due to a fear of rejection by partners and family, to fears of stigma and discrimination and/or to a tear of being blamed for the infection of others. It may also involve feelings of despair, remorse and guilt. Refusal to notify partners is very seldom due to a desire by the HIV-positive person to place another person deliberately at risk of HIV infection. For some, the consequences of their HIV status becoming known by their partners are severe. This is particularly the case for women who live in societies when women suffer social social, economic and legal disadvantages because they are women. In such places, a woman is often blamed for her own infection, as well as for the infection of her husband partner, oven though it is likely that she was infected by him. The reaction to disclosing her status may also include physical violence and abandonment, in which she (and her children) may be thrown out of the home and given no economic or social support. Thus, women may have very valid reasons for fearing to disclose their status to husbands/partners.

Given the possible serious consequences of counselling partners (discrimination, abandonment, violence) and of not counselling partners (transmission of HIV infection), counsellors and health care workers must be trained to handle the difficult ethical decisions to be made. In each case, all the potential harm and benefits of counselling or not counselling partners should be weighed. In most cases, with counselling and with a demonstration of support, the HIV-positive person will agree to notify partners. Initial support may take the form of notification in the presence of the counsellor and/or in the presence of another family member who will provide support and protection if necessary. Furthermore, there should be follow-up and referral to other support services to ensure that the couple or family can cope with the HIV-among them.

In cases where the source client refuses to notify, following repeated efforts to persuade him/her to do so, and where the failure to notify creates a clanger to a partner whose identity is known to the counsellor (in legal language "an identifiable risk to an identifiable third party"), the counsellor should be authorised to counsel the partner(s) without the consent of the source client.

In making this decision, the counsellor should ensure that the following factors are present.

- The HIV-positive person (source client) has been

thoroughly counselled as to the need for partner notification/counselling.

- The counselling has failed to achieve the appropriate behavioural changes, including the practice of safe sex.
- The source client has refused to notify, or consent to the counselling, of his/her partner(s).
- A real risk of HIV transmission to the identifiable partner(s) exists.
- The source client is given reasonable advance notice of the intention to counsel by the health care worker.
- The identity of the source client is concealed from the partner(s) if this is possible in practice.
- Follow-up is provided to ensure support to those involved as necessary and to prevent violence, family disruption etc. Recommendations for encouraging ethical partner counselling.

To encourage ethical partner counselling, UNAIDS and WHO recommend the following:

- Develop national policies and public health legislation on partner counselling that protect the principles of confidentiality and informed consent, and provide for the limited and clearly defined circumstances under which partner counselling may take place without consent.
- Develop public health legislation that authorises health care providers to decide, on the basis of each individual case and ethical considerations, whether to counsel partners without the consent of the source client, under certain circumstances.
- Hold consultations among health care providers,

government and affected communities about how to encourage ethical partner counselling and protect people who disclose their status through such counselling.

- Provide training and guidelines for health care providers and counsellors about how to protect confidentiality and informed consent in the context of partner counselling how to encourage and assist voluntary partner counselling: how to make difficult ethical decisions in cases where there is refusal to counsel partners and how to counsel partners in ways that harm is minimised and support is provided.
- Promote the establishment of professional ethical codes among health care and social service providers which require respect for confidentiality and informed constant in the context of partner counselling, and provide penalties for unethical conduct.
- Establish mechanisms for accountability and ways of making complaints in health care institutions and in communities when partners are counselled unethically by health care providers and other professionals.
- Support practical legal and social measures that address the vulnerability of people, particularly that of women to stigma, physical violence and abandonment, including projects in the community which will assist providing treatment, care, emotional support and protection from discrimination to those involved in partner counselling.

- Promote and support community projects about people's responsibility to protect themselves and others from HIV infection, particularly among men and boys.

Counselling on Sexuality

Sexuality is more than sexual behaviour and sexual intercourse. It includes social roles, personality, gender and sexual identity biology, relationships, thoughts and feelings. It has changing significance for people in various stages of life. Sexuality is affected by age, gender, culture and sexual orientation. The expressions of sexuality are influenced by various factors including social, ethical, economic, spiritual, cultural and moral concerns.

People find it difficult to talk about sexuality and often only accept it when there are important reasons, such as protection from STI and HIV. People need to accept their own sexuality and communicate about it if they are to-assess and reduce their risk of STI/HIV infection. Many clients would like to talk to their counsellor about their sexual relationships and intimacy. They may feel that this is the only person with whom they can share their feelings about sexual relationships and STI and HIV, without fear of discrimination.

The primary sexual attraction to the same, opposite or both sexes is termed as sexual orientation. Most societies find it hard to acknowledge and accept that homosexuality or be sexuality are a universal part of human sexuality. Many gays, lesbians or bisexuals neither experience nor desire a choice in their sexual orientation.

The sexual activities that people engage in are commonly called sexual behaviours. For example, a married man may have sex with men sometimes as well as his wife, but not identify himself as homosexual. Counselling aims to create a climate where all clients ran express themselves without fear of discrimination. All people, whatever their HIV status, have sexual feelings and may need help to feel able to express those sexual feelings safely and happily.

Sexual pleasure depends on *a* variety of factors, including mood, where and why people have sex and what society feels is appropriate or not appropriate behaviour. Sexual satisfaction rises when there is more intimacy between the partners. Understanding and accepting our own sexual desires and those of our partner helps to build intimacy, as well as being close in non-sexual ways. Cultures differ greatly in how they view different types of relationships and sexual activities. Women are usually expected to follow stated rules more than men. Everyone has the right to pursue sexual happiness in their own way, but only where the happiness and health of others is not at risk. Forced sex is wrong. No one has the right to have sex with a partner if it degrades her or him to an impersonal object. Everyone has the right to say no to sex at any time. Sexual pleasure need not be limited to sexual intercourse.

Unsafe sex might be very pleasurable for clients. Discuss safer sex not only in terms of STI, HIV and pregnancy prevention, but also explore ways to make safer sex pleasurable. Enable clients to talk about same sex activities or more than one sexual partner even if they are married. Do not make any assumptions about their sexual behaviour. Be aware that sex may not be pleasurable or consensual for the client. Explore the relationship between gender relations and sexual pleasure.

It is important for counsellors to be aware of how gender roles and stereotypes influence sexual relationships. The inequity between men and women is reflected in sexual relationships, making both women and men vulnerable to STI/ HIV. There are often double standards on sexual activity. Women are expected to abstain from sex before marriage and be faithful in marriage, whilst men are 'allowed' or expected to be sexually active before marriage and to have sexual relations outside marriage.

In many societies, men are socialised to treat women as interior in order to exercise power over them. Sexual acts do not always take place between two consenting adults, but involve domination of one person by another. Women and young people may not have the right to refuse sex if their partners or an older person asks for it. Disagreement over the use of preventive methods can lead to abusive situations. Men may feel that the prevention of unwanted pregnancies and even STI/HIV is a female concern. On the other hand, women who carry condoms or use contraceptives may be accused of promiscuity; This results in conflicts with men demanding unprotected sex but expecting women to protect themselves.

The sexual pleasure of men is often considered more important than that of women. Women are seen as providers and men as seekers of pleasure. Women may be accused of promiscuity if they ask for or obviously enjoy sex. Ignorance and lack of communication about sex may contribute to this problem. Men and women may not know about the importance of the clitoris for female pleasure or that women can have orgasms.

In some cultures, women are expected to have dry tight vaginas to please their partners. A sexually aroused women thought to be 'loose' or to have an STI. This practice puts them at risk of STI/HIV because the vagina wall easily tears and condoms are more likely to break. Some women undergo genital cutting, which can involve the removal of the clitoris and labia and closing of the opening to the vagina to a small hole. This makes sex painful and the trauma and bleeding put these women at higher risk of HIV. This practice is believed to preserve chastity and fidelity and gives men more control over women.

National laws may promote greater equity between men and women and positive sexual and reproductive health practices. These laws may be different from local norms related to culture, religion and class. The law may state that girls should not marry until they are 18 years old, but local culture promotes marrying girls after puberty to avoid premarital sex. Universal human rights and sexual and reproductive rights include the right to life and to bodily integrity and making our own decisions about sexual activity, marriage and having children.

How can counsellors help clients to empower themselves?

- Explore clients' opinions about gender inequalities in sexual life and challenge their
- Help clients to understand the impact of gender inequality on their sexual lives and health and look for ways to change them.
- Collaborate with other organisations and groups in the area who are working to change gender norms, improve gender relations and make them more equitable. Explore the origins of harmful practices with male and female clients, and their advantages and disadvantage. Challenge clients to have a new perspective on them.
- Educate clients about laws and universal rights and seek ways to put them into practice.

- Counsel men and women separately, in couples, and in small single sex or mixed groups so that they understand the views and feelings of the opposite sex. Show images of responsible, caring and assertive men and women.
- Provide information on male and female sexuality and sexual response to enhance mutual sexual pleasure. Include this in local ways of socialising young men and women on their gender and sexual roles.
- Help clients to know their rights and practice assertiveness and negotiation skills through role-play.

Counselling on Safer Sex, STI and HIV

Counselling on safer sex, STI and HIV helps clients to assess their own risks of HIV infection and STI in the past, now and in the future and to make a plan to reduce risks. It aims.

(i) To helps clients, whatever their HIV status, re-think their sexual lives and find ways to enjoy safer sex.

(ii) To help clients to feel positive about male/female condom use.

(iii) To identify clients who have a Reproductive Tract Infection (RTI) or STI so that they can receive prompt treatment and prevent (further infection in partners.

(iv) To help clients to take RTI/STI treatment correctly.

(v) To help clients with STI to inform, all their partners of the need to go for check up and treatment.

The counsellor has to find his own ways to introduce the topic of STI and HIV in a counselling session. If clients come and express concerns about HIV or STI, affirm their sense of responsibility and decision to take action. Assure them of confidentiality. Each client will have their particular needs so the counsellor has to give all clients an opportunity to discuss and get help on any aspect of their sexual lives. Many people wish to protect their fertility and have healthy children and one of the ways the counsellor can help clients do this is to protect themselves from STI/HIV. He may find it easier to begin to talk about the risk of STI/HIV when he is helping the clients to choose a contraceptive method. He could then begin a more in depth exploration of their risk and options for reducing it. If the client says nothing about HIV in a family planning counselling session, the counsellor might say something like:

"There is a lot of concern these days about HIV and AIDS. The counsellor can give all the clients an opportunity to discuss this issue with the counsellor so that they can think about their own lives and take any necessary action to stay safe. Would you like to do this?" If clients do not wish to talk about STI or HIV, the counsellor can to ensure that they are aware of the potential risk of STI and HIV and what they can do to reduce those risks. Encourage the clients to tell about any genital signs or symptoms that concern them.

Women are often too embarrassed to talk about genital problems. The counsellor need to ask: "Do you have any problems in your private parts that you would like to talk to me about? For example, vaginal discharge?" "Do you have any worries about illnesses passed through sex that you would like to talk to me about?" Offer visual screening for signs and symptoms of STI. Explain that some women do not show any signs or symptoms of STI but the germs can still be damaging their organs. Offer the client screening tests and explain the test procedure.

Counselling Client with an STI Diagnosis

In counselling client with an STI siagnosis the counsellor should follow the steps given below:

(i) Affirm the client and assure her or him of confidentially.

(ii) Encourage the client to tell you about any signs and symptoms, recent sexual interactions. fears and what they have already done to try to solve the problem.

(iii) Explain that the examination or test showed that they have an infection in their genitals passed through sexual intercourse. Explain and answer the client's question about it.

(iv) Explain that STIs can have serious consequences if the are not treated as quickly as possible. Explain the potential consequences of the client's particular STIs if they arc not treated.

(v) Explain that most STIs are curable if they are treated early with a complete course of the correct drugs. Explain about the prognosis for the clients STI. Stress the importance of taking the full occurs of correct drugs. Too little of the correct drug may make the infection difficulty to cure next time. Wrong drugs or local treatments may not kill all the pathogens or cure the infection.

(vi) If necessary, refer the client to the best local facility for, STI treatment and discuss any barriers he has to seeking treatment there. If he has concerns about issues such as travel, costs, attitudes of provides and confidentiality, look for ways to work with the service providers to improve the quality or certain exemption.

(vii) Explain what will happen at the health unit, when it opens and what the nurse will need to know and do.

(viii) Explain that clients need to tell all their sexual partners about the infection so that they get treatment. If women-have no symptoms and are would and treated, they may become very ill or infertile and they are at higher risk of HIV. Also, partners can re-infect each other every time they have sex if they are not both treated.

(ix) Generally it is difficult for women to tell men about STI infection because of gender inequality and men often do not wish to tell their partners. This is a serious problem which you can help to solve in collaboration community programmes.

(x) Explore the best way for clients to tell their partner the infection. Think about when, where, who it helps, role-play the best approach and timing the partner might react to the news and what the client could do to minimise risk of rejection, conflict or abuse.

(xi) If clients are anxious about telling their partners or are not able to do so, explore alternatives with them. Take great care not to push them into a potentially dangerous situation.

Partners may refuse to come for an STI test and/or treatment, especially if they do not have symptoms. They may wish to go to a different facility and/or take treatment without counselling or a test. Clients may refuse to tell their partners because they blame them or they want to keep their outside relationships secret. Some people lie to their stable partners about the nature of an STI. This may prevent quarrels but everyone has a right to information about their risk of STI/HIV. Understanding of the risks of infertility and damage to babies can motivate people to seek STI treatment promptly and to inform their partners. Understanding the increased risk of HIV and its impact on both clients and families can motivate a change of behaviour.

Group counselling for men can help to change attitudes. Both partners should abstain from sex until they are completely cured. If they are unable to do this, they should use condoms each time they have sex. Explain that STIs increase the risk of HIV. Stress the importance of prevention of STI and ask if clients wish to consider taking an HIV test.

If the client is in an ongoing relationship. STIs frequently result in conflicts because they imply that one or both parties have had a relationship outside. Women are often blamed, punished and rejected more than men, although their stable partner often infects them. Ask the client how she or he is feeling. Give her or him time to express their feelings about the situation.

While counselling a couple, give them a chance to say how they feel to each other while the other person really listens. Give positive examples of couples who have been in this situation and come through it and are still together. Help the couple to really listen and talk to each other about their thoughts and feelings to increase their understanding. Help them to talk about what they like sexually and what they can both do to avoid this problem in future. In this way, the counsellor have an opportunity to help the couple to talk more openly about what is going on in their sexual lives. Although this can be painful, it may finally help the relationship. While counselling one person, use role-play to practice communication.

Clients may need more support in talking to their partners, accessing and taking the correct treatment, and changing their own behaviour or that of their partners so they are not infected again. Arrange the next meeting to see whether they are cured and how their relationship is going. Find out whether they have been to the health unit, what medicine they are taking and whether the signs and symptoms have gone.

Counselling before HIV Antibody Testing

Counselling before HIV antibody testing aims to help the client to freely make an informed choice on whether or not to take the HIV antibody test on the basis of full and accurate information on the potential benefits and costs in their lives. The counsellor should find out what clients know about the HIV antibody test. Explain how the HIV antibody test works, the window period and the meaning of a positive, negative and uncertain result. Help clients to explore the advantages and disadvantages of taking the test in their own lives. Table 1 gives some ideas on this.

Never persuade or pressure clients to have an HIV antibody test. For any individual, the disadvantages of doing this may outweigh the advantages, particularly if testing facilities are poor or they are not in a powerful position in the family.

Counselling HIV Positive Clients

Telling clients that they have HIV infection is distressing and difficult for counsellor and client. If the client does not have AIDS, explain the difference between HIV and AIDS again and say that many people remain healthy for a long period of time with HIV infection.

Psychological support: The counsellor have a very important role in providing psychological support to clients and helping them to access support systems at home.

- Identify and explore clients'.
- Ask questions like "would you like to tell me more."
- Let clients know that their feelings are natural and that they are likely to change after the initial shock of learning the test result.
- Talk over again the questions you discussed during the pre-counselling session.
- Explore how clients were able to deal with other difficult situations in the past.
- Identify sources of support available to the client for example, family, friends, partner, church and clubs. Give the client any additional information about local sources of support, such as groups for People living with HIV/ or AIDS (PLWHA), church members and counselling organisations.
- Explore the client's ability to cope and ways of coping. These might include song, prayer, long walks, spending time with family and friends or joining a support group.
- If the client expresses any suicidal thoughts or ideas, take them seriously, even if the test is anonymous and confidential. Make sure that they have support before you see them next time.
- Assess the client's medical, preventive, and psychological support needs and discuss access to existing services.

Making a Plan

- Ask the client what they are planning to do when they leave the session and, if necessary, remind their, of the plan they made in the pro-test session for what they would do if their result was positive. Talk through the plan with them.
- Assess the client's social support and plans for partner notification.
- Help the client to establish, a plan for continuing medical. social and psychological support.
- Help clients to identify possible actions that may help resolve or ease their problems.
- Identify with clients task that they feel able to accomplish with the counsellor's support.
- Set up a follow-up session or refer as appropriate.

Counselling HIV Negative Clients

- Help clients to understand that a negative result only means that the test has not detected any antibodies. Help them to consider the possibility that they could be infected and not yet showing antibodies to HIV.
- Ask clients whether they have engaged in any risky sexual activity over the past three months. If they have, suggest that they avoid any risky sex from now on and have another test in three months time or longer. They should act as if they are HIV positive until they get the results of repeat test.
- Give all clients the opportunity to repeat the test to be sure of the result if they wish.

Counselling When the Test Result is Not Clear

Sometimes the results of the test do not tell whether

the test is positive or negative. This is frustrating for the client. This occurs rarely and may be because the person is in the pre-sero conversion phase. In this case, they should have a repeat test.

- Ask the client when they were last at risk of HIV infection Ask them to come for a repeat test three months or longer after this date.
- Explain that the client needs to take the same precaution for reducing risk as a person testing HIV positive until the time of the repeat test.

Counselling Sexually-abused Clients

Both women and men can suffer from abuse related to sex, but generally men abuse women. For this reason, let us refer to the abused person as 'she' and the abuser as 'he', whilst recognising that males may also be abused by other men or women.

There may be several type of abuses in a relationship. They are:

- *Physical abuse* involves physical assault. It includes hitting, punching, kicking, pulling hair and throwing things at someone. It can result in permanent injury disability and death. In most cases men use it to frighten women so that they can control them.
- *Sexual abuse* is where a person forces another to have sexual intercourse or other activities against their will inflicts pain during sex or does not allow the partner to use contraception or protection against STI/HIV. This can result in emotional trauma, illness and death..
- *Sexual harassment* includes making unwanted sexual comments, touches or propositions.

- *Psychological abuse* includes threats of suicide, violence or taking the children away, destruction of property or precious things or making a person perform degrading or dangerous acts.
- *Economic abuse* includes keeping partners short of money for basic needs, stopping her getting a job or forcing her to do sex work; controlling the money and spending it on his own desires; destruction of property and undermining partner's attempts to improve education.
- Economic exploitation includes manipulating someone to have sex they don't want with the offer of material rewards, jobs or basic needs.

Any of these forms of abuse can take place at home, in the workplace, in school, in public places or in religious institutions.

Sexual cultures and gender norms vary across ethnic groups and abuse, violence and coercion are viewed in different ways. In some cultures, married women are obliged to have sex with their husbands, whether they like it or not and rape in marriage does not exist in law; and men have a right to beat their wives if they step out of line. However, cultures are changing continuously and most countries have signed up to human rights agreements that everyone has a right to choice in sexual activity and to be protected from violence.

Counselling to Prevent Parent-to-Child Transmission of HIV/AIDS

HIV can be transmitted from an infected mother to her child during pregnancy, delivery and breast-feeding. Transmission ranges from 15-25 per cent in rich countries to 25-45 per cent in resource poor countries. The extra risk of HIV infection when an infant is breast-fed is around 15 per cent. There are a number of interventions that can reduce the risk of transmission to as low as 10 per cent. The health, well-being and sexuality of mothers as women is important, so counsel them on all the issues of safer sex when they attend services, not just pregnancy and preventing transmission to the child.

The prevention of HIV transmission to Pregnant Women, Mothers and their Children (PMTCT) includes:

- The prevention of HIV infection in women, mothers and mothers-to-be;
- The prevention of unwanted pregnancies;
- The prevention of HIV transmission from the infected mother to the infant.

The prevention of HIV in men and women of child-bearing age is a very important strategy for individuals, couples and communities as well as counsellors. Safe sexual behaviour and fast treatment of STI greatly reduces risk of transmission to children. Men have a major responsibility to practice safe sex and inform their female partners if they are at risk of STI. Women need awareness of the benefits of condoms and the ability to negotiate safer sex. Family planning counsellor's are key to the prevention of unwanted pregnancies. Making contraceptives, emergency contraception and safe abording accessible to all women, rich or poor, young or old, unmarried or single would reduce the rate of transmission to infants.

Prevention of transmission of HIV through pregnancy and breast-feeding involves: .

- STI screening and treatment;

- Accessible, high quality Voluntary Counselling. Testing (VCT) for mothers and fathers;
- Safe sex during pregnancy and breast-feeding;
- Prophylactic treatment by anti-retroviral drugs;
- Avoidance of invasive obstetrical procedures;
- Alternatives to early mixed feeding and prolonged feeding;
- Safe sex after delivery to-prevent unwanted Pregnancies.

These options require high quality ante-natal care (ANC) and VCT, care during delivery, post-natal care for mother and child and counselling on infant feeding. If VCT is promoted it is at ethical imperative to ensure that women who are HIV positive have access to long-term care and support. The advantage of VCT before, during and after delivery depend on the availability of treatment, the possibility of safer sex and support.

Counselling before Conception

Counselling before conception could include:

- Voluntary testing for one or both partners.
- Counselling on the positive and negative points in conceiving at this time.
- Counselling about reasons for wanting to conceive a baby when the woman and/or her partner is HIV positive.
- Minimising the risk of HIV transmission in becoming pregnant.

  Risks of mother to child transmission and options to prevent PMTCT.

- Increased risk of PMTCT if HIV contracted during pregnancy and breast-feeding.
- Long-term outcome for mother and baby, including ill-health, stigma and loss of parents.
- STI diagnosis and treatment.
- STI and HIV prevention in pregnancy, safer sex for both partners.
- Need to attend early for antenatal care to benefit fully.

Counselling Pregnant Women and Their Partners

Women at antenatal clinics have the same rights to informed consent and need the same pre-test counselling as clients in any other setting. Help them to think through the advantages and disadvantages of testing in relation to the baby as well as their own lives. Do not promote testing and be honest about the support that can offer if the result is positive.

Merits

- Know, understand and are helped to cope with HIV status.
- Empowered to make good choices about having or termination.
- Access to appropriate health care for mother and child.
- Access to information about negotiating for safer sex.
- Support with prevention of HIV transmission (for those testing negative and positive).
- To help partner share her HIV status.

- Gain access to ongoing support (social and emotional) through shared confidentiality.

Demerits

- Emotional distress.
- Stigma.
- Abuse or abandonment by partner.
- Breached confidentiality.
- Frustration if no treatment or support is available.

Counselling for HIV Positive Woman

Telling partners about the test result: It is often particularly difficult for a woman tested at the antenatal clinic to inform her partner she is positive soon after getting the result. Her partner and family may blame her for bringing the infection into the family although the status of her partner is unknown and he may have infected her. This can have a long-lasting negative impact on her psychosocial and economic well-being and family life. Testing at antenatal clinics can make, people see HIV and AIDS as a woman's disease. In some settings counselling and testing partners together is very helpful. In others, couples do not wish to be tested together. It is important to provide VCT in settings where men feel comfortable.

Counselling on continuation of pregnancy: Women who test HIV positive in early pregnancy in countries where abortion as safe and legal, may wish to discuss whether to continue the pregnancy or have a termination.

Methods to prevent mother to child transmission: Talk to clients about the available treatment and care options for prevention of Mother to Child Transmission so that they can make informed decisions relating to their pregnancy. If the counsellor can offer or refer for ARV treatments, informed consent, detailed explanations, monitoring and follow-up are particularly important, as the procedure is complex. It may involve a number of different services, including family planning and infant feeding support. It is essential that the client takes the drugs correctly. The counsellor can help the client to do this if he understands the regime, the risks and benefits.

Mothers who have ARV treatment should not breast-feed their infants because the drug goes into her breast milk and may harm the baby. The feasibility and safety of alternative infant feeding in the mother's particular circumstances may determine whether she decides to have ARV treatment. The number of infants of mothers receiving short course ARV treatment who contract HIV is greatly reduced to around. 10 per cent. These infected infants need continuing medical care and they, their mothers and families need social and emotional support.

REFERENCES

Academy for Educational Development, *Fundamental's of HIV Prevention Counselling: Participants Manual,* 1998.

"Candle of hope: the AIDS programme of the Thai Red Cross". *Strategies for Hope* Series, No. 9. London: Action Aid. 1994.

"Commodity Management in VCT Programmes: A Planning Guide". FHI/MSH-RPM, 2003.

Counselling for HIV / AIDS: a key to caring. For policy-makers, planners and implementors of counselling activities, Geneva: WHO. 1995.

Dhaliwal, Mandeep, et al., *Scaling up HIV Testing and Counselling Services a toolkit for programme managers.* International HIV/ AIDS Alliance, 2003.

Engender Health. *STI / HIV Prevention—Quick Reference Cards for*

Health Care Providers--What Every Client Should Known, New York, 2001.

Gordon, G. and Gordon, P., *Counselling and Sexuality: A Video Based Training Resource,* IPPF, London, 1992.

Government of India, *National AIDS Control Programme, HIV Testing Policy,* 1995.

Joint United Nations Programme on HIV/AIDS, *Counselling and HIV/AIDS: UNAIDS Technical Update,* November. 1997.

"Keys to Counselling", *AIDS Action Newsletter,* Issue 24. London AHRTAG. 1994.

Ndondo, Koziqhu. T., "Preventing mother-to-child transmission of HIV. A training manual for healthcare providers". *Reproductive Health Alliance.* London. 2001.

Programme guidance on Counselling for STI/HIV prevent in sexual and reproductive health settings. International Planned Parenthood Federation (IPPF), 2002.

Sittitrai W., *Reproductive health and HIV/AIDS. Myanmar training manual: a community-based approach for youth and women* Yangon. UNICEF, 1995.

South African AIDS Training (SAT) Programme, Basic counselling *guidelines in HIV and AIDS,* July, 2001.

The Bangkok Collaborative Perinatal HIV Transmission Study Group *Counselling Pregnant Women and New Mothers about HIV* Produced by the HIV/AIDS Collaboration, Thailand, 1999.

UNAIDS. *Counselling and voluntary HIV testing for pregnant women in high prevalence countries: Guidance for service providers* May, 1999.

UNAIDS policy on HIV testing and counselling. Geneva: UNAIDS 1997.

Voluntary Counselling and Testing (VCT): Program tools for implementing VCT, CDC, *Global AIDS Program,* April. 2003.

Welbourn, A.. "Stepping Stones: A Training Package (on HIV/AIDS communication and relationship skills, *Strategies for Hope* 1995."

Glossary

ACROMEGALY: A chronic disease caused by hypersecretion of the pituitary growth hormones. It is characterized by enlargement of many parts of the skeleton, especially the nose, ears, jaws, fingers and toes.

ACUTE INFECTION: An infection causing disease with a sudden onset, severity and (often) short course. As related to HIV infection: Once the virus enters the body, HIV infects a large number of CD4+ T cells and replicates rapidly. During this acute or primary phase of infection, the blood contains many viral particles that spread throughout the body, seeding themselves in various organs, particularly the lymphoid tissues.

ACUTE RETROVIRAL SYNDROME: The acute or primary HIV infection often passes unrecognized, but may be present as a mononucleosis-like syndrome within three months of the infection. The diagnosis is made by demonstrating HIV antibody seroconversion.

ACYCLOVIR: (Acycloguanosine). A nucleoside analog antiviral drug used to treat the symptoms of the genital form of herpes simplex virus infection. S

ADENOPATHY: Any disease involving or causing enlargement of glandular tissues, especially one involving the lymph nodes.

ADJUVANT: An ingredient-as in a prescription or solution-that facilitates or modifies the action of the principal ingredient. May be used in HIV therapies or for HIV vaccines.

ADMINISTRATION: (Route of Administration). A term used to refer to how a drug or therapy is introduced into the body. Systemic administration means that the drug goes throughout the body (usually carried in the bloodstream), and includes oral administration (by mouth) and intravenous administration (injection into the vein). Local administration means that the drug is applied or introduced into the specific area affected by the disease, such as application directly onto the affected skin surface (topical administration). The effects of most therapies depend upon the ability of the drug to reach the affected area, thus the route of administration and consequent distribution of a drug in the body is an important determinant of its effectiveness.

ADVERSE EVENT: In a clinical trial, an unwanted effect detected in participants. The term is used whether or not the effect can be attributed to the intervention under study.

AEROSOLIZED: A form of administration in which a drug, such as pentamidine, is turned into a fine spray or mist by a nebulizer and inhaled.

AFFECTED COMMUNITY: This includes HIV-positive people, persons living with AIDS and other individuals, including their families, friends and advocates, directly impacted by HIV infection and its physical, psychological and sociological ramifications.

AGAMMAGLOBULINEMIA: A nearly total absence of immunoglobulins.

AGENCY FOR HEALTH CARE POLICY AND RESEARCH (AHCPR): An agency of the Public Health Service that supports activities to enhance health care services and improve access to them.

AIDS BIBLIOGRAPHY: The National Library of Medicine publishes the monthly AIDS Bibliography, which includes all citations from the AIDSLINE database. The AIDS Bibliography is available from the Superintendent of Documents.

AIDS CLINICAL TRIALS GROUP (ACTG): The ACTG is composed of a number of US medical centers that valuate treatment for HIV and HIV-associated infections. ACTG studies are sponsored by the National Institute of Allergy and Infectious Diseases.

AIDS DEMENTIA COMPLEX: About half the people infected with HIV, the virus that causes AIDS, develop infections or other problems involving the brain or spinal cord. These neurological complications may include inflammation of the brain (encephalitis), or of the membrane surrounding the brain (meningitis), infections of the brain, brain or spinal cord tumors, nerve damage, difficulties in thinking and behavioral changes (i.e., AIDS dementia complex) and stroke.

AIDSDRUGS: An online database service administered by the National Library of Medicine, with references to drugs undergoing testing against AIDS, AIDS-related complex and related opportunistic infections.

AIDS EDUCATION AND TRAINING CENTERS (AETC): The Health Resources and Services Administration supports a network of 15 regional centers that serve as resources for educating health professionals in prevention, diagnosis and care of HIV-infected patients. The centers train primary caregivers to incorporate HIV prevention strategies into their clinical priorities, along with diagnosis, counseling and care of HIV-infected persons and their families.

AIDS KNOWLEDGE BASE: Full-text electronic database on AIDS, available in print as well as electronic form, produced and maintained by physicians and other health care professionals. The database is edited by P.T. Cohen (San Francisco General Hospital), Merle Sande, and Paul Volberding.

AIDSLINE: An online database service administered by the National Library of Medicine, with citations and abstracts covering the published scientific and medical literature on AIDS and related topics.

AIDS-RELATED CANCERS: Several cancers are more common or more aggressive in people infected with HIV, the virus that causes AIDS. These malignancies include certain types of immune system cancers known as lymphomas, Kaposi's sarcoma and anogenital cancers primarily affecting the cervix and the anus. HIV, or the immune suppression it induces, appears to play a role in the development of these cancers.

AIDS-RELATED COMPLEX (ARC): 1. A term, not officially defined or recognized by the Centers for Disease Control and Prevention, that has been used to describe a variety of symptoms and signs found in some persons infected with HIV. These may include recurrent fevers, unexplained weight loss, swollen lymph nodes, and/or fungus infection of the mouth and throat. Also commonly described as symptomatic HIV infection. 2. Symptoms that appear to be related to infection by the HIV virus. They include an unexplained, chronic deficiency of white blood cells (leukopenia) or a poorly functioning lymphatic system with swelling of the lymph nodes (lymphadenopathy) lasting for more than three months without the opportunistic infections required for a diagnosis of AIDS.

AIDS RESEARCH ADVISORY COMMITTEE: Board that advises and makes recommendations to the Director, National Institute of Allergy and Infectious Diseases, on all aspects of HIV-related research, vaccine development, pathogenesis and epidemiology.

AIDS SERVICE ORGANIZATION (ASO): A health

association, support agency or other service active in the prevention and treatment of AIDS.

AIDSTRIALS: An online database service administered by the National Library of Medicine, with information about clinical trials of agents under evaluation against HIV infection, AIDS and related opportunistic infections.

ALKALINE PHOSPHATASE: An enzyme that is normally present in certain cells within the liver, bone, kidney, intestine and placenta. When the cells are destroyed in those tissues, more of the enzyme leaks into the blood, and levels rise in proportion to the severity of the condition. Measurement of this enzyme is used as an indication of the health of the liver.

ALOPECIA: The loss of hair that frequently occurs in patients undergoing chemotherapy for cancer or suffering from other diseases, such as AIDS, where cell-killing, or cytotoxic, drugs are used.

ALTERNATIVE THERAPY: In Western countries, alternative therapy refers to any type of medicine that supplements or is used in lieu of biomedicine (i.e., conventional medicine) or allopathic medicine. In other parts of the world, where traditional medicine predominates, the term may refer to biomedicine itself.

ALUM: Potassium aluminum sulfate or ammonium aluminum sulfate, used especially as an emetic (i.e., an agent that induces vomiting), an astringent (i.e., a substance that contracts tissues) and styptic (i.e., a substance that tends to check bleeding by contracting the tissues or blood vessels).

ALVEOLAR: Pertaining to the alveoli sac, the site of gas exchange in the lungs.

AMEBIASIS: An inflammation of the intestines caused by infestation with Entameba histolytica (a type of ameba) and characterized by frequent, loose stools flecked with blood and mucus.

AMINO ACIDS: Any of a class of organic compounds having a carboxyl group (COOH) and an amino group (NH2). Some 22 amino acids are commonly found in animals, and more than 100 less common forms are found in nature, chiefly in plants. When the carboxyl carbon atom of one amino acid binds to the nitrogen of another with the release of a water molecule, a linkage called a peptide bond is formed. Chains of amino acids, joined head-to-tail in this manner, are synthesized by living systems and are called polypeptides (up to about 50 amino acids) and proteins (over 50 amino acids).

AMNIOCENTESIS: The surgical insertion of a hollow needle through the abdominal wall and into the uterus of a pregnant female to obtain amniotic fluid (i.e., the serous fluid in which the embryo is suspended) especially to examine the fetal chromosomes for an abnormality or for the determination of the sex of the embryo.

ANALOG: In chemistry, a compound with a structure similar to that of another compound, but differing from it in respect to certain components or structural makeup; it may have a similar or opposite action metabolically.

ANAMNESTIC RESPONSE: The heightened immunologic reaction elicited by a second or subsequent exposure to a particular pathogenic microorganism or antigen.

ANAPHYLACTIC SHOCK: A life-threatening allergic reaction characterized by a swelling of body tissues (including the throat) and a sudden decline in blood pressure.

ANERGY: 1. The loss or weakening of the body's immunity to an irritating agent, or antigen. The strength of the body's immune response is often quantitatively measured by means of a skin test where a solution containing an antigen known to cause a response, such as mumps or candida, is injected immediately under the skin. The lack of a reaction to these common antigens indicates anergy. 2. Researchers in cell culture have shown that

CD4+T cells can be turned off by a signal from HIV that leaves them unable to respond to further immune system stimulation. This inactivated state is known as anergy.

ANTIBIOTIC: An antimicrobial agent, derived from cultures of a microorganism or produced semisynthetically, used to treat infections.

ANTIBODIES: Molecules in the blood or secretory fluids that tag, destroy or neutralize bacteria, viruses or other harmful toxins. They are members of a class of proteins known as immunoglobulins, which are produced and secreted by B lymphocytes in response to stimulation by antigens. An antibody is specific to an antigen.

ANTIFOLATE: An agent that inhibits intracellular (i.e., inside cells) production of folinic acid.

ANTIGEN: A substance that, when introduced into the body, is capable of inducing the production of a specific antibody. es.

ANTIIDIOTYPE: An antibody that recognizes and binds to another antibody (idiotype).

ANTINEOPLASTIC: Inhibiting or preventing the proliferation of tumor cells.

ANTIRETROVIRAL AGENTS: Substances used against retroviruses such as HIV.

ANTITOXINS: Antibodies that recognize and inactivate toxins produced by certain bacteria, plants or animals.

ANTIVIRAL: A substance or process that destroys a virus or suppresses its replication.

APOPTOSIS: Cellular suicide, also known as programmed cell death. HIV may induce apoptosis in both infected and uninfected immune system cells. Uninfected cells may also undergo apoptosis. Normally when CD4+ T cells mature in the thymus gland, a small proportion of these cells are unable to distinguish self from nonself. Because these cells would otherwise attack the body's own tissues, they receive a biochemical signal from other cells that results in apoptosis.

ARM: A group of participants in a clinical trial, all of whom receive the same treatment or placebo.

ASPERGILLOSIS: A fungal infection (resulting from the fungus Aspergillus) of the lungs that can spread through the blood to other organs. Symptoms include fever, chills, difficulty in breathing and coughing up blood. If the infection reaches the brain, it may cause dementia.

ASSEMBLY AND BUDDING: Names for a portion of the processes by which new HIV virus is formed in infected host cells. Viral core proteins, enzymes and RNA (ribonucleic acid) gather just inside the cell's membrane, while the viral envelope proteins aggregate within the membrane. An immature viral particle is formed and then pinches off from the cell, acquiring an envelope and the cellular and HIV proteins from the cell membrane. The immature viral particle then undergoes processing by an HIV enzyme called protease to become an infectious virus.

ASYMPTOMATIC: Without symptoms. Usually used in AIDS literature to describe a person who has a positive reaction to one of several tests for HIV antibodies, but who shows no clinical symptoms of the disease.

ATTENUATED: Weakened or decreased. For example, an attenuated virus can no longer produce disease, but might be used to produce a vaccine.

AUTOANTIBODY: 1. An antibody that is active against some of the tissues of the organism that produced it. 2. An antibody directed against the body's own tissue.

AUTOIMMUNIZATION: The induction in an individual of an immune response to its own cells (tissue).

AUTOINOCULABLE: Susceptible of being inoculated with microorganisms from one's own body.

AUTOLOGOUS: Pertaining to the same organism or one of its parts; originating within an organism itself.

AZT: Azidothymidine (also called zidovudine or ZDV; the Burroughs-Wellcome trade name is Retrovir). One of the first drugs used against HIV infection, AZT is a nucleoside analog that suppresses replication of HIV.

BACTERIOSTATIC: Capable of inhibiting reproduction of bacteria.

BACTERIUM: A microscopic organism composed of a single cell. Many bacteria can cause disease in humans.

BACULOVIRUS: A virus of insects used in the production of some HIV vaccines.

BASELINE: 1. Information gathered at the beginning of a study from which variations found in the study are measured. 2. A known value or quantity with which an unknown is compared when measured or assessed.

BASOPHIL: A type of white blood cell, also called a granular leukocyte, filled with granules of toxic chemicals that can digest microorganisms. Basophils, as well as other types of white blood cells, are responsible for the symptoms of allergy. The granules stain blue when exposed to a basic dye for microscopic examination.

BILIRUBIN: 1. A bile pigment whose measurement can be used as an indication of the health of the liver. 2. A substance released from old or damaged red blood cells. Small amounts of bilirubin normally enter the bloodstream and circulate until they reach the liver and then into the bowel, where bilirubin is further broken down and excreted. The normal value is 0.1 to 1.5 milligrams per liter of blood.

BINDING ANTIBODY: As related to HIV infection: An antibody that attaches to some part of the HIV virus. Binding antibodies may or may not adversely affect the virus.

BIOLOGICAL RESPONSE MODIFIERS (BRMs): Substances, either natural or synthesized, that boost, direct or restore normal immune defenses. BRMs include interferons, interleukins, thymus hormones and monoclonal antibodies.

BIOPSY: The surgical removal of a piece of tissue from a living subject for microscopic examination to make a diagnosis (for example, to determine whether abnormal cells such as cancer cells are present).

BIOTECHNOLOGY: 1. The use of living organisms or their products to make or modify a substance. These include recombinant DNA techniques (also referred to as genetic engineering) and hybridoma technology. 2. The industrial application of the results of biological research, particularly in fields such as recombinant DNA or gene splicing, which permits the production of synthetic hormones or enzymes by combining genetic material from different species.

BLINDED STUDY: A clinical trial in which participants are unaware as to whether or not they are in the experimental or control arm of the study.

BLOOD BRAIN BARRIER: The barrier between brain blood vessels and brain tissues whose effect is to restrict what may pass from the blood into the brain.

B LYMPHOCYTES (B CELLS): One of the two major classes of lymphocytes. During infections, these cells are transformed into plasma cells that produce large quantities of antibody directed at specific pathogens. This transformation occurs through interactions with various types of T cells and other components of the immune system. In persons with AIDS, the functional ability of both the B and the T lymphocytes is damaged, with the T lymphocytes being the principal site of infection by the HIV virus.

BODY FLUIDS: Any fluid in the human body, such as blood, urine, saliva, sputum (spit), tears, semen, mother's milk or vaginal secretions. Only blood, semen, mother's milk and vaginal secretions have been linked directly to the transmission of the HIV virus.

BONE MARROW: Soft tissue located in the cavities of the bones where blood cells such as erythrocytes, leukocytes and platelets are formed.

BOOSTER: A second or later dose of a vaccine given to increase the immune response to the original dose.

BRANCHED DNA ASSAY: A sensitive, rapid test that can be used to monitor the amount of HIV in a patient's bloodstream (i.e., the viral burden).

BREAKTHROUGH INFECTION: An infection, caused by the infectious agent the vaccine is designed to protect against, that occurs during the course of a vaccine trial. These infections may be caused by exposure to the infectious agent before the vaccine has taken effect, or before all doses of the vaccine have been given. Breakthrough infections also occur in trial participants receiving placebos.

BRONCHOSCOPY: Visual examination of the bronchial passages of the lungs through a tube of an endoscope inserted into the upper lungs or extraction of material from the lungs by means of a bronchoscope.

BURKITT'S LYMPHOMA: A lymphatic cancer that involves not only the lymphatic and the associated reticuloendothelial system, but also other body tissues. This disease, which is most common in Central Africa, is thought to be possibly caused by the Epstein-Barr virus. Also called African lymphoma, Burkitt's tumor.

CACHEXIA: General ill health and malnutrition, marked by weakness and emaciation, usually associated with serious disease.

CANDIDA: Yeast-like fungi commonly found in the normal flora of the mouth, skin, intestinal tract and vagina, but can become clinically infectious in immune compromised people.

CANDIDIASIS: An infection with a fungus of the Candida family, generally Candida albicans; it most commonly involves the skin (dermatocandidiasis), oral mucosa (thrush), respiratory tract (bronchocandidiasis) and vagina (vaginitis). Candidiasis of the esophagus, trachea, bronchi or lungs is an indicator disease for AIDS.

CARCINOGEN: Any cancer-producing substance.

CATHETER: A tubular medical device for insertion into canals, vessels, passageways or body cavities, usually to permit injection (e.g., through an intravenous catheter into a vein) or withdrawal of fluids, or to keep a passage open.

CD8 (T8) CELLS: A protein embedded in the cell surface of suppressor T lymphocytes. Also called cytotoxic T cells.

CD4 (T4) or CD4+ CELLS: 1. White blood cells killed or disabled during HIV infection. These cells normally orchestrate the immune response, signaling other cells in the immune system to perform their special functions. Also known as T helper cells. 2. HIV's preferred targets are cells that have a docking molecule called cluster designation 4 (CD4) on their surfaces. Cells with this molecule are known as CD4-positive (or CD4+) cells. Destruction of CD4+ lymphocytes is the major cause of the immunodeficiency observed in AIDS, and decreasing CD4+ lymphocyte levels appear to be the best indicator of morbidity in these patients. Although CD4 counts fall, the total T-cell level remains fairly constant through the course of HIV disease, due to a concomitant increase in the CD8+ cells. The ratio of CD4+ to CD8+ cells is therefore an important measure of disease progression.

CDC NATIONAL AIDS CLEARINGHOUSE: The CDC's comprehensive reference, referral and publication distribution service for HIV and AIDS information. The Clearinghouse works in partnership with national, regional, state and local organizations that develop and deliver HIV prevention programs and services.

CD NOMENCLATURE: This nomenclature was developed to standardize and compare monoclonal antibodies from different sources. Antibodies with similar reactivity patterns are assigned to CD groups representing "clusters of differentiation." T lymphocytes are CD3+ and can be separated into the CD4+ T helper cells and the CD8+ cytotoxic/suppressor cells. Although CD4+ cells are predominantly T lymphocytes, some monocytes are also CD4+.

CELL LINES: Specific cell types artificially maintained in the laboratory (i.e., in vitro) for scientific purposes.

CELL-MEDIATED IMMUNITY (CMI): The branch of the immune system in which the reaction to foreign material is performed by specific defense cells (i.e., killer cells, macrophage and other white blood cells) rather than antibodies.

CENTERS FOR DISEASE CONTROL AND PREVENTION (CDC): A Public Health Service agency responsible (among others) for assessing the status and characteristics of the AIDS epidemic and the prevalence of HIV infections. CDC supports the design, implementation and evaluation of prevention activities, and maintains various HIV/AIDS information services, such as the CDC National AIDS Clearinghouse.

CENTRAL NERVOUS SYSTEM (CNS): Composed of the brain, spinal cord and its coverings (meninges).

CENTRAL NERVOUS SYSTEM (CNS) DAMAGE: (By HIV infection). Although monocytes and macrophages can be infected by HIV, they appear to be relatively resistant to killing. However, these cells travel throughout the body and carry HIV to various organs, especially the lungs and the brain. People infected with HIV often experience abnormalities in the central nervous system. Investigators have hypothesized that an accumulation of HIV in brain and nerve cells or the inappropriate release of cytokines or toxic byproducts by these cells may be to blame for the neurological manifestations of HIV disease.

CERVICAL CANCER: A neoplasm of the uterine cervix that can be detected in the early curable stage by the Papanicolaou (Pap) test.

CERVICAL DYSPLASIA: A precursor lesion for cervical cancer. Studies indicate an increase in prevalence of cervical dysplasia among HIV-infected women. Additional studies have documented that a higher prevalence is associated with greater immuno suppression. HIV infection also may adversely affect the clinical course and treatment of cervical dysplasia and cancer.

CERVICAL INTRAEPITHELIAL NEOPLASIA (CIN1, CIN2, CIN3): Dysplasia of the cervix epithelium, often pre-malignant (i.e., cancerous), characterized by various degrees of hyperplasia, abnormal keratinization (forming horny epidermal tissue) and condylomata. Considerable evidence implicates human papilloma virus (HPV) in the development of CIN. Immunosuppression may also play an important role in facilitating infection or persistence of HPV in the genital tract and progression of HPV-induced neoplasia.

CERVIX: The part of the uterus that protrudes into the cavity of the vagina.

CHALLENGE: In vaccine experiments, the exposure of an immunized animal to the infectious agent.

CHEMOTHERAPY: The treatment, mostly of cancer, by the use of a series of cytotoxic drugs that attack cancerous cells. This treatment commonly has adverse side effects that may include the temporary loss of the body's natural immunity to infections, loss of hair, digestive upset and a general feeling of illness. Although unpleasant, the adverse effects of treatment are tolerated considering the life-threatening nature of the cancers usually treated by chemotherapy.

CLINICAL: Pertaining to or founded on observation and treatment of patients, as distinguished from theoretical or basic science.

CLINICAL ALERT: A mechanism, adopted by the National Institutes of Health in onjunction with the editors of several biomedical journals, for urgent cases in which timely and broad dissemination of results of clinical trials could prevent morbidity (sickness) and mortality (death). The Clinical Alert does not become a barrier to subsequent publication of the full research paper. Clinical Alerts are widely distributed electronically through the National Library of Medicine and through standard mailings.

CLINICAL LATENCY: The state or period of an infectious agent, such as a virus or bacterium, living or developing in a host without producing clinical symptoms. As related to HIV infection: Although infected individuals usually exhibit a period of clinical latency with little evidence of disease, the virus is never truly latent. Even early in the disease, HIV is active within lymphoid organs where large amounts of virus become trapped in the FDC network. Surrounding germinal centers are areas rich in CD4+ T cells. These cells increasingly become infected and viral particles accumulate both in infected cells and as free virus.

CLINICAL PRACTICE GUIDELINES: Standards for physicians to adhere to in prescribing care for a given condition or illness.

CLINICAL TRIAL: A carefully designed and executed investigation of the effects of a drug (or vaccine) administered to human subjects. The goal is to define the clinical efficacy and pharmacological effects (toxicity, side effects, incompatibilities or interactions) of the drug. The US government, through the Food and Drug Administration, requires strict testing of all new drugs and vaccines prior to their approval for use as therapeutic agents.

COCCIDIOIDOMYCOSIS: An infectious fungal disease caused by the inhalation of spores of Coccidioides immitis, which is carried on windblown dust particles. The disease is endemic in hot dry regions of the Southwestern US and Central and South America, and is an opportunistic disease associated with AIDS. Also called desert fever, San Joaquin fever, valleyfever.

COMMUNITY-BASED CLINICAL TRIAL (CBCT): A clinical trial conducted primarily through primary-care physicians rather than academic research facilities.

COMMUNITY-BASED ORGANIZATION (CBO): A locally based service organization that provides social services at the community level.

COMMUNITY PROGRAMS FOR CLINICAL RESEARCH ON AIDS (CPCRA): An initiative of the National Institute of Allergy and Infectious Diseases (NIAID) to broaden the base of clinical investigations by involving community physicians in AIDS research and trials. NIAID started the CPCRA in 1989. It is one of four HIV clinical trials programs supported by NIAID. In 1992 the name of the program was officially changed to the Terry Beirn Community Programs for Clinical Research on AIDS.

COMPASSIONATE USE: A method of providing experimental drugs to very sick patients who have no other treatment options. Often, case-by-case approval must be obtained from the Food and Drug Administration for "compassionate use" of a drug.

COMPLEMENT: A group of proteins in normal blood serum and plasma which, in combination with antibodies, causes the destruction of antigens, particularly bacteria and foreign blood corpuscles.

COMPLEMENT CASCADE: A precise sequence of events, usually triggered by an antigen-antibody complex, in which each component of the complement system is activated in turn.

CONCOMITANT DRUGS: Drugs that are taken together. Certain concomitant medications may have adverse interactions.

CONCORDE STUDY: Joint French/British clinical trial of AZT in asymptomatic HIV-positive individuals.

CONDYLOMA: (Condyloma acuminatum). A papilloma with a central core of connective tissue in a treelike structure covered with epithelium, usually occurring on the mucous membrane or skin of the external genitals or in the perianal (tissue surrounding the anus) region. Although the lesions are usually few in number, they may aggregate to form large cauliflower-like masses. Caused by the human papilloma virus (HPV), it is infectious and autoinoculable (i.e., capable of being transmitted by inoculation from one part of the body to another). Also called acuminate or venereal warts.

CONTAGIOUS: Any infectious disease capable of being transmitted by casual contact from one person to another. Casual contact can be defined as normal day-to-day contact between people at home, school, work or in the community. A contagious infection (e.g., a common cold) can be communicable by casual contact; an infectious infection, on the other hand, is communicable by intimate contact such as sex. AIDS is infectious, not contagious.

CONTRAINDICATION: A specific circumstance when the use of certain treatments could be harmful.

CONTROL: A standard against which experimental observations may be evaluated. In clinical trials, one group of patients is given an experimental drug, while another group (i.e., the control group) is given either a standard treatment for the disease or a placebo.

CORE PROTEIN: As related to HIV: An integral protein of the HIV virus composed of three units, p24, p15 and p18.

CORRELATES OF IMMUNITY/CORRELATES OF PORTECTION: The immune responses that protect an individual from a certain disease. The precise identities of the correlates of immunity in HIV are unknown.

CREATININE: A protein found in muscles and blood, and excreted by the kidneys in the urine. The level of creatinine in the blood and urine provides a measure of kidney function.

CRYPTOCOCCAL MENINGITIS: A life-threatening infection of the membranes (meninges) that line the brain and the spinal cord. Cryptococcal disease is caused by a fungus (Cryptococcus neoformans). Most people have been exposed to this organism, which is found in soil contaminated by bird droppings, but it usually does not cause disease in healthy people. The majority of people with cryptococcal meningitis have immune systems that are damaged by disease, such as AIDS, or suppressed by drugs. The organism can infect almost all organs of the body, although it most commonly causes disease of the meninges, skin or lungs.

CRYPTOCOCCOSIS: An infectious disease seen in HIV-infected patients due to the fungus Cryptococcus neoformans, which is acquired via the respiratory tract. It can spread from the lungs to the brain, the central nervous system, the skin, skeletal system and urinary tract.

CRYPTOSPORIDIOSIS: An opportunistic infection caused by the protozoan parasite Cryptosporidium parvum.

CT: (Computed Tomography). Radiography (using X-rays) in which a three-dimensional image of a body structure is constructed by computer from a series of plane cross-sectional images made along an axis. Also referred to as CAT scan.

CYTOMEGALOVIRUS (CMV): A herpes virus that is a common cause of opportunistic diseases in people with AIDS and other people with immune suppression. While CMV can infect most organs of the body, people with

AIDS are most susceptible to CMV retinitis (disease of the eye) and colitis (disease of the colon

CYTOMEGALOVIRUS (CMV) RETINITIS: Most adults in the US have been infected by cytomegalovirus, although the virus usually does not cause disease in healthy people. Because the virus remains in the body for life, it can cause disease if the immune system becomes severely damaged by disease or suppressed by drugs. CMV retinitis is an eye disease common among people who are infected with HIV. Without treatment, people with CMV retinitis can lose their vision. CMV infection can affect both eyes and is the most common cause of blindness among people with AIDS.

CYTOTOXIC T LYMPHOCYTE (CTL): A lymphocyte that is able to kill foreign cells that have been marked for destruction by the cellular immune system.

DATA SAFETY AND MONITORING BOARD (DSMB): An independent committee, composed of community representatives and clinical research experts, that reviews data while a clinical trial is in progress to ensure that participants are not exposed to undue risk. A DSMB may recommend that a trial be stopped if there are safety concerns or if the trial objectives have been achieved.

DDC: Dideoxycytidine (zalcitabine, HIVID), a nucleoside analog drug that inhibits the replication of HIV.

DDI: Dideoxyinosine (didanosine, Videx), a nucleoside analog drug that inhibits the replication of HIV.

DELETION: Elimination of a gene (i.e., from a chromosome) either in nature or in the laboratory.

DEMENTIA: Chronic intellectual impairment (i.e., loss of mental capacity) with organic origins that affects a person's ability to function in a social or occupational setting.

DEMYELINATION: Destruction, removal or loss of the myelin sheath of a nerve or nerves.

DENDRITE: Any of the usual branching protoplasmic processes that conduct impulses toward the body of a nerve cell.

DENDRITIC CELLS: Patrolling immune system cells that may begin the HIV disease process by carrying the virus from the site of the infection to the lymph nodes, where other immune cells become infected. Dendritic cells travel through the body and bind to foreign invaders-such as HIV-especially in external tissues, such as the skin and the membranes of the gut, lungs and reproductive tract. They then ferry the foreign substance to the lymph nodes to stimulate T cells and initiate an immune response. In laboratory experiments, the dendritic cells that carry HIV also bind to CD4+ T cells, thereby allowing HIV to infect the CD4+ T cells. CD4+ T cells are the critical immune system cells targeted by HIV and depleted during HIV infection.

D4T: (Also known as Stavudine and Zerit). d4T is a dideoxynucleoside pyrimidine analog (2'3'-didehydro-3'-deoxythymidine). Like other nucleoside analogs, d4T inhibits HIV replication by inducing premature viral DNA chain termination. d4T has been approved for patients with advanced HIV infection intolerant to or failing other antiretroviral drugs.

DIAGNOSIS: The determination of the presence of a specific disease or infection, usually accomplished by evaluating clinical symptoms and laboratory tests.

DIARRHEA: Uncontrolled, loose and frequent bowel movements. In the United States, almost all people with AIDS develop diarrhea at some time in the course of their disease. Severe or prolonged diarrhea can lead to weight loss and malnutrition. The excessive loss of fluid that may occur with AIDS-related diarrhea can be life-threatening. There are many possible causes of diarrhea in people who have AIDS. The most common infectious organism causing AIDS-related diarrhea include cytomegalovirus (CMV); the parasites Cryptosporidium, Microsporidia and Giardia lamblia; and the bacterium Mycobacterium avium-inracellulare (MAC). Other bacteria and parasites that cause diarrheal symptoms in otherwise healthy people may cause more severe, prolonged or recurrent diarrhea in people with HIV or AIDS.

DNA: (Deoxyribonucleic Acid). 1. The molecular chain found in genes within the nucleus of each cell, which carries the genetic information that enables cells to reproduce. 2. DNA is the principal constituent of chromosomes, the structures that transmit hereditary characteristics. The amount of DNA is constant for all typical cells of any given species of plant or animal (including humans), regardless of the size or function of that cell. Each DNA molecule is a long, two-stranded chain made up of subunits, called nucleotides, containing a sugar (deoxyribose), a phosphate group and one of four nitrogenous bases: adenine (A), guanine (G), thymine (T) and cytosine (C). In 1953 J.D. Watson and F.H. Crick proposed that the strands, connected by hydrogen bonds between the bases, were coiled in a double helix. Adenine bonds only with thymine (A-T or T-A) and guanine only with cytosine (G-C or C-G). The complementarity of this bonding ensures that DNA can be replicated (i.e., that identical copies can be made in order to transmit genetic information to the next generation).

DOSE-RANGING STUDY: A clinical trial in which two or more doses of an agent (such as a drug) are tested against each other to determine which dose works best and is least harmful.

DRUG-DRUG INTERACTION: A modification of the effect of a drug when administered with another drug. The effect may be an increase or a decrease in the action of either substance, or it may be an adverse effect that is not normally associated with either drug.

DYSPLASIA: Any abnormal development of tissues or organs. In pathology, alteration in size, shape and organization of adult cells.

ELISA: (Enzyme-Linked Immunosorbent Assay). A laboratory test to determine the presence of antibodies to HIV in the blood. A positive ELISA test generally is confirmed by the Western Blot test.

END-STAGE DISEASE: Final period or phase in the course of a disease leading to a person's death.

ENV: A gene of HIV that codes for the protein gp160, the precursor of the envelope proteins gp120 and gp41.

ENVELOPE: In virology, a protein covering that packages the virus's genetic information. The outer coat, or envelope, of HIV is composed of two layers of fat-like molecules called lipids taken from the membranes of human cells. Embedded in the envelope are numerous cellular protein, as well as mushroom-shaped HIV proteins that protrude from the surface. Each mushroom is thought to consist of a cap made of four glycoprotein molecules called gp120 and a stem consisting of four gp41 molecules embedded in the envelope. The virus uses these proteins to attach to and infect cells.

ENZYME: A protein that accelerates a specific chemical reaction without altering itself (i.e., a catalyst).

EOSINOPHIL: A type of white blood cell, called granulocyte, that can digest microorganisms. The granules can be stained by the acid dye, eosin, for microscopic examination.

EPIDEMIC: A disease that spreads rapidly through a demographic segment of the human population, such as everyone in a given geographic area, a military base, or similar population unit, or everyone of a certain age or sex, such as the children or women of a region. Epidemic diseases can be spread from person to person or from a contaminated source such as food or water.

EPIDEMIOLOGIC SURVEILLANCE: The ongoing and systematic collection, analysis and interpretation of data about a disease or health condition. As part of a surveillance system to monitor the HIV epidemic in the US, the CDC, in collaboration with state and local health departments, other federal agencies, blood collection agencies and medical research institutions, conducts standardized HIV seroprevalence surveys in designated subgroups in the US population. Collecting blood samples for the purpose of surveillance is called serosurveillance.

EPIDEMIOLOGY: The branch of medical science that deals with the incidence, distribution and control of a disease in a population.

EPITHELIUM: The covering of the internal and external organs of the body. Also the lining of vessels, body cavities, glands and organs. It consists of cells bound together by connective material and varies in the number of layers and the kinds of cells.

EPITOPE: A unique shape or marker carried on an antigen's surface that triggers a corresponding antibody response.

EPSTEON-BARR VIRUS (EBV): A herpes-like virus that causes one of the two kinds of mononucleosis (the other is caused by CMV). It infects the nose and throat and is contagious. EBV lies dormant in the lymph glands and has been associated with Burkitt's lymphoma and hairy leukoplakia.

ERYTHEMA: Redness or inflammation of the skin or mucous membranes.

ERYTHEMA MULTIFORME: A skin disease characterized by papular (small, solid, usually conic elevation of the skin) or vesicular lesions (blisters), and reddening or discoloration of the skin often in concentric zones about the lesion. Erythema multiforme has been associated with many infections, collagen disease, drug sensitivities, allergies and pregnancy. A severe form of this condition is Stevens-Johnson Syndrome.

ERYTHROCYTES: Red blood cells whose major function is to carry oxygen to cells.

ETIOLOGY: The study or theory of the factors that cause disease.

EXCLUSION/INCLUSION CRITERIA: The medical or social standards determining whether a person may or may not be allowed to enter a clinical trial. For example, some trials may not include people with chronic liver disease, or may exclude people with certain drug allergies; others may exclude men or women or only include people with a lowered T-cell count.

EXPANDED ACCESS: A general term for methods of distributing experimental drugs to patients who are unable to participate in ongoing clinical trials and have no other treatment options. Specific types of expanded access mechanisms include parallel track, Treatment IND, and compassionate use.

FALLOPIAN TUBES: Part of the female reproductive system. A pair of ducts opening at one end into the uterus and at the other end into the peritoneal cavity, over the ovary. Each tube serves as a passage through which the ovum (egg) is carried to the uterus and through which spermatozoa (sperm) move toward the ovary.

FOLIC ACID: A crystalline vitamin of the B complex that is used especially in the treatment of nutritional anemias. It occurs in green plants, fresh fruit, liver and yeast. Also called folacin, folate, vitamin B9.

FOLINIC ACID: Also called citrovorum factor. A metabolically active form of folic acid that has been used in cancer therapy to protect normal cells against methotrexate (a cancer chemotherapy agent). Also used to treat megaloblastic anemias.

FOLLICLE: A small anatomical cavity or deep narrow-mouthed depression; a small lymph node.

FOLLICULAR DENDRITIC CELLS (FDCs): Cells found in the germinal centers of lymphoid organs. FDCs have thread-like tentacles that form a weblike network to trap invaders and present them to other cells of the immune system (for destruction).

FOMITE: An inanimate object that can harbor pathogenic microorganisms and thus serve as an agent of transmission of an infection.

FOOD AND DRUG ADMINISTRATION (FDA): The Public Health Service agency responsible for (among others) ensuring the safety and effectiveness of drugs, biologics, vaccines and medical devices used in the diagnosis, treatment and prevention of HIV infection, AIDS and AIDS-related opportunistic infections. The FDA also works with the blood banking industry to safeguard the nation's blood supply.

FUNCTIONAL ANTIBODY: An antibody that binds to an antigen and has an effect. For example, neutralizing antibodies inactivate HIV or prevent it from infecting other cells.

FUNGUS: 1. A general term used to denote a class of microbes including mushrooms, yeasts and molds. 2. Fungi, which were once classified as plants, have since been reclassified as unmoving organisms that lack chlorophyll. Mycologists (scientists working with fungi) estimate that there are 100,000 species of fungi, ranging from baker's yeast to dermatophytes (fungi that cause ringworm and athlete's foot) to potentially invasive species such as Candida albicans and Aspergillus. As many as 150 of these organisms have now been linked to animal or human diseases.

GANGLION: A mass of nervous tissue, composed principally of nerve-cell bodies, usually lying outside the central nervous system.

GASTROINTESTINAL: Relating to the stomach and intestines.

GENE: 1. Ultimate unit by which inheritable characteristics are transmitted to succeeding generations in all living organisms. Genes are contained by, and arranged along the length of, the chromosome. The gene is composed of deoxyribonucleic acid (DNA). Each chromosome of each species has a definite number and arrangement of genes, which govern both the structure and metabolic functions of the cells and thus of the entire organism. They provide information for the synthesis of enzymes and other proteins and specify when these substances are to be made. Alteration of either gene number or arrangement can result in mutation (a change in the inheritable traits). 2. A unit of DNA that carries information for the biosynthesis of a specific product (in the cell).

GENETIC ENGINEERING: Group of new research techniques that manipulate the DNA (genetic material) of cells. The gene-splicing technique, which produces recombinant DNA, is a method of transporting selected genes from one species to another. For example, in this technique, the genes, which are actually portions of molecules of DNA, are removed from the donor (insect, plant, mammal or other organism) and spliced into the genetic material of a virus; then the virus is allowed to infect recipient bacteria. In this way the bacteria become recipients of both viral and foreign genetic material. When the virus replicates within the bacteria, large quantities of the foreign as well as viral material are made.

GENITOURINARY TRACT: The system of organs comprising the organs concerned with the production and excretion of urine and those concerned with reproduction. Also called genitourinary system, urogenital system, urogenital tract.

GENOME: The complete set of genes in the chromosomes of each cell of a particular organism.

GERMINAL CENTERS: Structures within lymphoid tissues that contain FDCs in which immune responses are initiated.

GIARDIASIS: A common protozoal infection of the small intestine spread via contaminated food and water and direct person-to-person contact.

GLYCOPROTEIN: A conjugated protein in which the nonprotein group is a carbohydrate (i.e., a sugar molecule); also called glucoprotein.

GP41: Glycoprotein 41, a protein embedded in the outer envelope of HIV. Plays a key role in HIV's infection of CD4+ T cells by facilitating the fusion of the viral and the cell membranes.

GP120: Glycoprotein 120, a protein that protrudes from the surface of HIV and binds to CD4+ T cells.

GP160: Glycoprotein 160, a precursor of HIV envelope proteins gp41 and gp120.

GRANULOCYTE: A cell type of the immune system filled with granules of toxic chemicals that enable them to digest microorganisms. Basophils, neutrophils, and eosinophils are examples of granulocytes.

HALF-LIFE: The time required for half the amount of a drug to be eliminated from the body.

HEALTH RESOURCES AND SERVICES ADMINISTRATION (HRSA): A Public Health Service agency that administers (among others) education and training programs for health care providers and community service workers who care for AIDS patients. HRSA also administers programs to demonstrate how communities can organize their health care resources to develop an integrated, comprehensive system of care for those with AIDS and HIV infection.

HELPER/SUPPRESSOR RATIO: (Of T cells). T cells are lymphocytes (white blood cells) that are formed in the thymus and are part of the immune system; they have been found to be abnormal in people with AIDS. The normal ratio of helper T cells (CD4+ cells) to suppressor T cells (CD8+ cells) is approximately 2:1. This becomes inverted in people with AIDS, but may be abnormal for a host of other temporary reasons.

HEMATOCRIT: A laboratory measurement that determines the percentage of packed red blood cells in a given volume of blood.

HEMATOTOXIC: Poisonous to the blood or bone marrow.

HEMOGLOBIN: The component of red blood cells that carries oxygen.

HEPATITIS: An inflammation of the liver caused by certain viruses and other factors such as alcohol abuse, some medications and trauma. Although many cases of hepatitis are not a serious threat to health, the disease can become chronic and can sometimes lead to liver failure and death. There are four major types of viral hepatitis: (a) hepatitis A, caused by infection with the hepatitis A virus; (b) hepatitis B, caused by infection with the hepatitis B virus (HBV), which is most commonly passed on to a partner during intercourse, especially during anal sex, as well as through sharing drug needles; (c) non-A, non-B hepatitis, caused by the hepatitis C virus, which appears to be spread through sexual contact as well as through sharing drug needles (another type of non-A, non-B hepatitis is caused by the hepatitis E virus, principally spread through contaminated water) (d) delta hepatitis occurs only in people who are already infected with HBV and is caused by the HDV virus; most cases of delta hepatitis occur among people who are frequently exposed to blood and blood products such as people with hemophilia.

HERPES SIMPLEX VIRUS I (HSV-I): A virus that causes

cold sores or fever blisters on the mouth or around the eyes, and can be transmitted to the genital region. The latent virus can be reactivated by stress, trauma, other infections or suppression of the immune system.

HERPES SIMPLEX VIRUS II (HSV-II): A virus causing painful sores of the anus or genitals that may lie dormant in nerve tissue. It can be reactivated to produce the symptoms. HSV-II may be transmitted to a neonate (newborn child) during birth from an infected mother, causing retardation and/or other serious complications. HSV-II is a precursor of cervical cancer.

HERPES VARICELLA ZOSTER VIRUS: The varicella virus causes chicken pox in children and may reappear in adults as herpes zoster. Also called shingles, herpes zoster consists of very painful blisters on the skin that follow nerve pathways.

HISTOCOMPATIBILITY TESTING: A method of matching the self antigens on the tissues of a transplant donor with those of a recipient. The closer the match, the better the chance that the transplant will not be rejected.

HISTOPLASMOSIS: A fungal infection, commonly of the lungs, caused by the fungus Histoplasma capsulatum. This fungus is commonly found in bird and/or bat droppings in the Ohio and Mississippi Valley region, the Caribbean Islands and in parts of the Northeast US. It is spread by breathing in the spores of the fungus. The most definitive test for the fungus has been from fungal stains and bone marrow cultures. Blood testing has proved to be less reliable. In areas where H. capsulatum is prevalent, 80 percent or more of the population has been exposed to infection through breathing in airborne spores produced by the fungus. People with severely damaged immune systems, such as those with AIDS, are vulnerable to a very serious disease known as progressive disseminated histoplasmosis. Nationwide, about 5 percent of people with AIDS have histoplasmosis, but in geographic areas where the fungus is common, people with AIDS are at high risk for disseminated histoplasmosis.

HIV DISEASE: Characterized by a gradual deterioration of immune function. During the course of infection, crucial immune cells called CD4+ T cells are disabled and killed, and their numbers progressively decline. CD4+ T cells play a crucial role in the immune response, signaling other cells in the immune system to perform their special functions.

HOMOLOGOUS: Similar in appearance or structure, but not necessarily function.

HOST: A plant or animal harboring another organism.

HOST FACTORS: The body's potent mechanisms for containing HIV, including immune system cells called CD8+ T cells, which may prove more effective than any antiretro-viral drug in controlling HIV infection.

HUMAN IMMUNODEFICIENCY VIRUS TYPE 1 (HIV-1): 1. The retrovirus isolated and recognized as the etiologic (i.e., causing or contributing to the cause of a disease) agent of AIDS. HIV-1 is classified as a lentivirus in a subgroup of retroviruses.

HUMAN IMMUNODEFICIENCY VIRUS TYPE 2 (HIV-2): A virus closely related to HIV-1 that has been found to cause immune suppression. Most commonin Africa.

HUMAN LEUKOCYTE ANITGENS (HLA): Markers that identify cells as "self" and prevent the immune system from attacking them.

HUMAN PAPILLOMA VIRUS (HPV): A virus that is the cause of warts of the hands and feet, as well as lesions of the mucous membranes of the oral, anal and genital cavities. More than 50 types of HPV have been identified, some of which are associated with cancerous and precancerous conditions. The virus can be transmitted through sexual contact and is a precursor to cancer of the cervix. There is no specific cure for an HPV infection, but the virus often can be controlled by podophyllin (medicine derived from the roots of the plant Podophyllum peltatum) or interferon, and the warts can be removed by cryosurgery, laser treatment or conventional surgery.

HUMORAL IMMUNITY: The branch of the immune system that relies primarily on antibodies.

HYBRID: An offspring produced from mating plants or animals from different species, varieties or genotypes.

HYBRIDOMA: A hybrid cell produced by the fusion of an antibody-producing lymphocyte with a tumor cell. Hybridomas are used in the production of monoclonal antibodies.

HYPERPLASIA: Abnormal increase in the elements composing a part (as tissue cells).

HYPOGAMMAGLOBULINEMIA: Abnormally low levels of immunoglobulins.

HYPOTHESIS: A tentative statement or supposition that may then be tested through research.

IDIOTYPES: The unique and characteristic parts of an antibody's variable region, which can themselves serve as antigens.

IMMUNE COMPLEX: Clusters formed when antigens and antibodies bind together.

IMMUNE DEFICIENCY: A breakdown or inability of certain parts of the immune system to function, thus making a person susceptible to certain diseases that they would not ordinarily develop.

IMMUNE RESPONSE: The activity of the immune system against foreign substances.

IMMUNE SYSTEM: The complex functions of the body that recognize foreign agents or substances, neutralize them and recall the response later when confronted with the same challenge.

IMMUNE THROMBOCYTOPENIC PURPURA (ITP): Also Idiopathic Immune Thrombocytopenic Purpura. A condition in which the body produces antibodies against the platelets in the blood, which are cells responsible for blood clotting. ITP is very common in HIV-infected people.

IMMUNITY: A natural or acquired resistance to a specific disease. Im-munity may be partial or complete, long-lasting or temporary.

IMMUNOCOMPETENT: 1. Capable of developing an immune response. 2. Possessing a normal immune system.

IMMUNOGEN: A substance, also called an antigen, capable of provoking an immune response.

IMMUNOGENICITY: The ability of an antigen or vaccine to stimulate an immune response.

IMMUNOMODULATOR: Any substance that influences the immune system.

IMMUNOSTIMULANT: Any agent or substance that triggers or enhances the body's defense; also called immunopotentiators.

IMMUNOSUPPRESSION: A state of the body in which the immune system is damaged and does not perform its normal functions. Immunosuppression may be induced by drugs or result from certain disease processes, such as HIV infection.

IMMUNOTHERAPY: Treatment aimed at reconstituting an impaired immune system.

IMMUNOTOXIN: A plant or animal toxin (i.e., poison) that is attached to a monoclonal antibody and used to destroy a specific target cell.

INCIDENCE: The number of new cases occurring in a given population over a certain period of time.

INCLUSION/EXCLUSION CRITERIA: The medical or social standards determining whether a person may or may not be allowed to enter a clinical trial. For example, some trials may not allow people with chronic liver disease or with certain drug allergies; others may exclude men or women, or only include people with a lowered T-cell count.

INCUBATION PERIOD: The time interval between the initial exposure to infection and appearance of the first symptom or sign of disease.

INDIAN HEALTH SERVICE (IHS): A Public Health Service agency providing a comprehensive health service delivery system for American Indians and Alaska Natives.

INFECTION: The state or condition in which the body (or part of the body) is invaded by an infectious agent (e.g., a bacterium, fungus or virus), which multiplies and produces an injurious effect (active infection). As related to HIV: Infection typically begins when HIV encounters a CD4+ cell. The HIV surface protein gp120 binds tightly to the CD4 molecule on the cell's surface. The membranes of the virus and the cell fuse, a process governed by gp41, another surface protein. The viral core, containing HIV's RNA, proteins and enzymes, is released into the cell. See CD4 (T4) or CD4+ Cells; gp41; gp120.

INFECTIOUS: Capable of being transmitted by infection, with or without actual contact.

INFORMED CONSENT: Type of protection available to people considering entering a drug trial. Before entering the trial, participants must sign a consent form that contains an explanation of: (a) why the research is being done, (b) what researchers want to accomplish, (c) what will be done during the trial and for how long, (d) what risks are in the trial, (e) what benefits can be expected from the trial, (f) what other treatments are available, and (g) the participant's right to leave the trial at any time.

INOCULATION: The introduction of a substance (inoculum; e.g., a vaccine, serum or virus) into the body to produce or to increase immunity to the disease or condition associated with the substance.

INSTITUTIONAL REVIEW BOARD (IRB): 1. A committee of physicians, statisticians, community advocates and others that ensures that a clinical trial is ethical and that the rights of study participants are protected. All clinical trials in the United States must be approved by an IRB before they begin.

INTEGRASE: An HIV enzyme used by the virus to integrate its genetic material into the host cell's DNA.

INTEGRATION: The process by which the different parts of an organism are made a functional and structural whole, especially through the activity of the nervous system and of hormones. As related to HIV: The process by which the viral DNA migrates to the cell's nucleus, where it is spliced into the host's DNA with the help of viral integrase. Once incorporated, HIV DNA is called the provirus and is duplicated together with the cell's genes every time the cell divides. Recent reports suggest that HIV's DNA also can integrate into the DNA of nondividing cells such as macro-phages and brain and nerve cells.

INTENT TO TREAT: Analysis of clinical trial results that includes all data from patients in the groups to which they were randomized (i.e., assigned through random distribution) even if they never received the treatment.

INTERFERON: A general term used to describe a family of 20-25 proteins that cause a cell to become resistant to a wide variety of viruses. They are produced by cells infected by almost any virus.

INTERLEUKIN-2 (IL-2): One of a family of molecules that control the growth and function of many types of lymphocytes. Interleukin-2 is an immune system protein produced in the body by T cells. It has potent effects on the proliferation, differentiation and activity of a number of immune system cells, including T cells, B cells and natural killer cells. Commercially, IL-2 is produced by recombinant DNA technology and is approved by the

Food and Drug Administration for the treatment of metastatic renal (i.e., kidney) cell cancer. Studies have shown that in the test tube, addition of IL-2 can improve some of the immunologic functions that are abnormal in HIV-infected patients. In addition, IL-2 is a growth factor for T cells, causing them to increase in number. In a clinical study with IL-2, it was found that in a small number of HIV-infected patients, IL-2 boosted levels of CD4+ T cells (i.e., the infection-fighting white blood cells normally destroyed during HIV infection) for more than two years, a far longer time than typically seen with currently available anti-HIV drugs.

INTRAVENOUS (IV): Of or pertaining to the inside of a vein, as of a thrombus, or an injection, infusion or catheter.

INTRAVITREAL: Within the eye.

INVESTIGATIONAL NEW DRUG (IND): The status of an experimental drug after the Food and Drug Administration agrees that it can be tested in people.

IN VITRO: ("In glass"). An artificial environment created outside a living organism (e.g., a test tube or culture plate) used in experimental research to study a disease or process.

IN VIVO: ("In life"). Studies conducted within a living organism (e.g., animal or human studies).

ISOLATE: An individual (as a spore or a single organism), viable part of an organism (as a cell) or a strain that has been isolated (as from diseased tissue, contaminated water or the air). Also, a pure culture produced from such an isolate. A particular strain of HIV taken from a patient.

KARNOFSKY SCORE: A subjective score between 0-100, assigned by a physician to describe a patient's ability to perform common tasks.

KILLER T CELLS: Killer cells infected with HIV or other viruses or transformed by cancer. Also known as cytotoxic T cells (or cytotoxic T lymphocytes).

LAI: A group of closely related HIV isolates that includes the LAV, IIIB and BRU strains of HIV. Used in HIV vaccine development.

LAK CELLS: Lymphocytes transformed in the laboratory into lymphokine activated killer cells, which attack tumor cells.

LANGERHANS CELLS: Dendritic cells in the skin that pick up an antigen and transport it to the lymph nodes.

LATENCY: The period when an organism (i.e., a virus or a bacterium) is in the body and not producing any ill effects.

LAV: Lymphadenopathy Associated Virus (see Human Immunodeficiency Virus Type I).

LENTIVIRUS: "Slow" virus characterized by a long interval between infection and the onset of symptoms. HIV is a lentivirus as is the simian immunodeficiency virus (SIV), which infects nonhuman primates.

LESION: A general term to describe an area of altered tissue (e.g., the infected patch or sore in a skin disease).

LEUKOPENIA: A decrease in the number of white blood cells. The threshold value for leukopenia is usually taken as less than 5000 white blood cells per cubic millimeter of blood.

LIPID: Any of a group of fats and fat-like compounds, including sterols, fatty acids and many other substances.

LONG TERMINAL REPEAT SEQUENCE (LTR): A component of the AIDS genome.

LONG-TERM NON-PROGRESSORS: Individuals who are HIV-infected for seven or more years, have stable CD4+ T cell counts of 600 or more cells per cubic millimeter of blood, no HIV-related diseases and no previous antiretroviral therapy. Data suggest that this phenomenon is associated with the maintenance of the integrity of the lymphoid tissues and with less virus-trapping in the lymph nodes than seen in other HIV-infected individuals.

LUMBAR: Of, relating to or constituting the loins or the vertebrae between the thoracic vertebrae and the sacrum region. The sacrum is the triangular bone made up of five fused vertebrae and forming the posterior section of the pelvis. The thorax is the part of the human body between the neck and the diaphragm, partially encased by the ribs and containing the heart and lungs; the chest.

LUMBAR PUNCTURE: A procedure in which fluid from the subarachnoid space in the lumbar region is tapped for examination. Also known as spinal tap.

LYMPH: A transparent, slightly yellow fluid that carries lymphocytes. Lymph is derived from tissue fluids collected from all parts of the body and is returned to the blood via lymphatic vessels.

LYMPHADENOPATHY SYNDROME (LAS): Swollen, firm and possibly tender lymph nodes. The cause may range from an infection such as HIV, the flu, mononucleosis or lymphoma (cancer of the lymph nodes).

LYMPHATIC VESSELS: A bodywide network of channels, similar to the blood vessels, that transport lymph to the immune organs and into the bloodstream.

LYMPH NODES: Small, bean-sized organs of the immune system, distributed widely throughout the body. Lymph fluid is filtered through the lymph nodes in which all types of lymphocytes take up temporary residence. Antigens that enter the body find their way into lymph or blood and are filtered out by the lymph nodes or spleen respectively, for attack by the immune system.

LYMPHOCYTE: A white blood cell. Present in the blood, lymph and lymphoid tissue.

LYMPHOID INTERSTITIAL PNEUMONITIS (LIP): A form of pneumonia that involves the lower lobes (of the lungs) with extensive alveolar infiltration by mature lymphocytes, plasma cells and histiocytes. LIP is associated with AIDS, dysproteinemia and other conditions.

LYMPHOID ORGANS: Include tonsils, adenoids, lymph nodes, spleen and other tissues. Act as the body's filtering system, trapping invaders(i.e., foreign particles from bacteria, viruses, etc.) and presenting them to squadrons of immune cells that congregate there. Within these lymphoid tissues, immune activity is concentrated in regions called germinal centers, where the thread-like tentacles of follicular dendritic cells (FDCs) form networks that trap invaders.

LYMPHOKINES: 1. Products of the lymphatic cells that stimulate the production of disease-fighting agents and the activities of other lymphatic cells. Among the lymphokines are gamma interferon and interleukin-2.

LYMPHOMA: Cancer of the lymphoid tissues. Lymphomas are often described as being large or small cell types, cleaved or noncleaved, diffuse or nodular. The different types often have different prognoses (i.e., prospect of survival or recovery). Some of these lymphomas are named after the physicians who first described them (e.g., Burkitt's lymphoma, Hodgkin's disease). Lymphomas can also be referred to by the organ where they are active such as CNS lymphomas, which are in the central nervous system, and GI lymphomas, which are in the gastrointestinal tract. The types of lymphomas most commonly associated with HIV infection are called non-Hodgkin's lymphomas or B cell lymphomas. In these types of cancers, certain cells of the lymphatic system grow abnormally. They divide rapidly, growing into tumors.

MAGNETIC RESONANCE IMAGING (MRI): Medical imaging that uses radiofrequency radiation as its source. MRI is a noninvasive diagnostic technique that can provide information on the form and function of internal tissues and organs of the body.

MAJOR HISTOCOMPATIBILITY COMPLEX (MHC): A group of genes that control aspects of the immune response. The products of these genes, the histocompatibility antigens, are present on every cell of the body and serve as markers to distinguish self from nonself cells.

MALABSORPTION SYNDROME: Decreased intestinal absorption resulting in loss of appetite, muscle pain and weight loss.

MALAISE: A generalized, nonspecific feeling of discomfort.

MAST CELL: A granulocyte found in tissue. The contents of the mast cells, along with those of basophils, are responsible for the symptoms of allergy.

MEAN: The arithmetic average, or the sum of all the values divided by the number of values.

MEDIAN: The middle number in a sequence of numbers, taken as the average of the two middle numbers when the sequence has an even number of numbers (e.g., 4 is the median of 1, 3, 4, 8, 9).

MEMORY CELLS: A subset of T lymphocytes that have been exposed to specific antigens and can then proliferate (i.e., reproduce) on subsequent immune system encounters with the same antigen.

MESSENGER RNA: Also referred to as mRNA. An RNA (ribonucleic acid) that carries the genetic code for a particular protein from the nuclear DNA (i.e., the DNA in the cell's nucleus) to a ribosome in the cytoplasm and acts as a template, or pattern, for the formation of that protein.

METABOLISM: The sum of the processes by which a particular substance is handled (as by assimilation and incorporation, or by detoxification and excretion) in the living body.

METABOLITE: Any substance produced by metabolism or by a metabolic process.

METASTASIS: Transfer of a disease-producing agent (e.g., cancer cells or bacteria) from an original site of disease to another part of the body with development of a similar lesion in the new location (e.g., spread of cancer from an original site to other sites in the body).

MICROBES: Microscopic living organisms, including bacteria, protozoa and fungi.

MICROBICIDE: An agent (e.g., a chemical or antibiotic) that destroys microbes.

MICROENCAPSULATED: Surrounded by a thin layer of protection. A means of protecting a drug or vaccine from rapid breakdown.

MICROSPORIDIOSIS: Disease resulting from infection with a protozoal pathogen from the Microsporida order.

MN: A strain of HIV used in vaccine development.

MOLECULE: The smallest particle of a compound that has all the chemical properties of that compound. Molecules are made up of two or more atoms, either of the same element or of two or more different elements. Ionic compounds, such as common salt, are made up not of molecules, but of ions arranged in a crystalline structure. Unlike ions, molecules carry no electrical charge. Molecules differ in size and molecular weight as well as in structure.

MOLLUSCUM CONTAGIOSUM: A disease of the skin and mucous membranes caused by a poxvirus. It is characterized by scattered flesh-toned white papules. The disease most frequently occurs in children and adults with impaired immune response. It is transmitted from person to person by direct or indirect contact and lasts up to three years.

MONOCLONAL ANTIBODIES: Antibodies produced by a hybridoma or antibody-producing cell source for a specific antigen. Monoclonal antibodies are useful as a tool for identifying specific protein molecules.

MONOVALENT VACCINE: A vaccine that is specific for only one antigen. See also Antigen.

MUCOCUTANEOUS: Anything that concerns or pertains to mucous membranes and the skin (e.g., mouth, vagina, lips, anal area).

MUCOSAL IMMUNITY: Resistance to infection across the mucous membranes. Dependent on immune cells and antibodies present in the lining of the urogenital tract, gastrointestinal tract and other parts of the body exposed to the outside world. See also Antibodies; Genitourinary Tract; Mucous Membrane.

MUCOUS MEMBRANE: A moist layer of tissue that lines body cavities or passages that have an opening to the external world (e.g., the lining of the mouth, nostrils or vagina).

MUTATION: In biology, a sudden change in a gene or unit of hereditary material that results in a new inheritable characteristic. In higher animals and many higher plants, a mutation may be transmitted to future generations only if it occurs in germ-or sex cell-tissue; body cell mutations cannot be inherited. Changes within the chemical structure of single genes may be induced by exposure to radiation, temperature extremes and certain chemicals. The term mutation may also be used to include losses or rearrangements of segments of chromosomes, the long strands of genes. Drugs such as colchicine double the normal number of chromosomes in a cell by interfering with cell division. Mutation, which can establish new traits in a population, is important in evolution. As related to HIV: HIV mutates rapidly. During the course of HIV disease, viral strains may emerge in an infected individual that differ widely in their ability to infect and kill different cell types, as well as in their rate of replication. Strains of HIV from patients with advanced disease appear to be more virulent and infect more cell types than strains obtained earlier from the same individual. See also Gene.

MYCOBACTERIUM AVIUM COMPLEX (MAC): 1. A common opportunistic infection caused by two very similar mycobacterial organisms, Mycobacterium avium and Mycobacterium intracellulare. 2. A bacterial infection that can be localized (limited to a specific organ or area of the body) or disseminated throughout the body. It is a life-threatening disease, although new therapies offer promise for both prevention and treatment. MAC disease is extremely rare in people who are not infected with HIV. See also Opportunistic Infection.

MYELIN: A substance that sheathes nerve cells, acting as an electric insulator that facilitates the conduction of nerve impulses.

MYELOSUPPRESSION: Impairment of the blood cell-producing function of the bone marrow.

NATIONAL CANCER INSTITUTE (NCI): An NIH institute with the overall mission of conducting and supporting research, training and disseminating health information with respect to the causes, diagnosis and treatment of cancer. NCI also performs these functions for HIV infections and associated diseases. See also National Institutes of Health.

NATIONAL INSTITUTE OF ALLERGY AND INFECTIOUS DISEASES (NIAID): An NIH institute that conducts and supports research to study the causes of allergic, immunologic and infectious diseases, and to develop better means of preventing, diagnosing and treating illnesses. NIAID is responsible for the federally funded, national basic research program in AIDS. See also National Institutes of Health.

NATIONAL INSTITUTE OF CHILD HEALTH AND HUMAN DEVELOPMENT (NICHD): An NIH institute that conducts and supports research on the reproductive, developmental and behavioral processes that determine the health of children, adults, families and populations. Thus, NICHD supports clinical research related to the transmission of HIV from infected mothers to their offspring, the progression of disease in HIV-infected infants and children, and the testing of potential therapies and preventatives for this population. See also National Institutes of Health.

NATIONAL INSTITUTES OF HEALTH (NIH): A multi-institute agency of the Public Health Service, NIH is the federal focal point for health research. It conducts research in its own laboratories and supports research in universities, medical schools, hospitals and research institutions throughout this country and abroad. See also Public Health Service.

NATIONAL LIBRARY OF MEDICINE (NLM): An NIH institute, NLM is one of three US national libraries. It is the world's largest research library in a single scientific and professional field (i.e., medicine). NLM provides (among others) electronic and print information services relating to HIV/AIDS, including AIDSLINE, AIDSTRIALS, AIDSDRUGS and the AIDS Bibliography. See also AIDS Bibliography; AIDSDRUGS; AIDSLINE; AIDSTRIALS; National Institutes of Health.

NATURAL HISTORY STUDY: Study of the natural development of something (such as an organism or a disease) over a period of time.

NATURAL KILLER CELLS: (NK cells). A type of lymphocyte that does not carry the markers to be B cells or T cells. Like cytotoxic T cells, they attack and kill tumor cells and protect against a wide variety of infectious microbes. They are "natural" killers because they do not need additional stimulation or need to recognize a specific antigen in order to attack and kill. Persons with immunodeficiences such as those caused by HIV infection have a decrease in "natural" killer cell activity. See also Antigen; B Lymphocytes; Cytotoxic; Lymphocyte; Null Cell; T Cells.

NECROLYSIS: Shedding of surface components of tissue, such as cells from internal body surfaces, due to death of a portion of tissue.

NEF: One of the regulatory genes of the HIV virus. Three HIV regulatory genes-tat, rev and nef-and three so-called auxiliary genes-vif, vpr and vpu-contain information necessary for the production of proteins that control the virus's ability to infect a cell, produce new copies of the virus or cause disease. See also rev; tat.

NEURALGIA: A sharp, shooting pain along a nerve pathway.

NEUROPATHY: The name given to a group of disorders involving nerves. Symptoms range from a tingling sensation or numbness in the toes and fingers to paralysis. It is estimated that 35 percent of people with HIV disease have some form of neuropathy. A "peripheral neuropathy" refers to the peripheral nerves outside the spinal cord.

NEUTRALIZATION: The process by which an antibody binds to specific antigens, thereby "neutralizing" the microorganism. See also Antibodies; Antigen.

NEUTRALIZING ANTIBODY: An antibody that keeps a virus from infecting a cell, usually by blocking receptors on the cell or the virus. See also Antibodies; Receptor.

NEUTRALIZING DOMAIN: The section of the HIV envelope protein gp120 that elicits antibodies with neutralizing activities. See also Antibodies; gp120.

NEUTROPENIA: An abnormal decrease in the number of neutrophils (the most common type of white blood cells) in the blood. The decrease may be relative or absolute. Neutropenia is associated with acute leukemia, infection, rheumatoid arthritis and other conditions.

NEUTROPHIL: Also called polymorphonuclear neutrophil (PMN). A white blood cell that plays a central role in defense of a host against infection. Neutrophils engulf and kill foreign microorganisms.

NSAID: Nonsteroidal anti-inflammatory (i.e., counteracting inflammation) drug.

NUCLEIC ACID: Organic substance, found in all living cells, in which the hereditary information is stored and from which it can be transferred. Nucleic acid molecules are long chains that generally occur in combination with proteins. The two chief types are DNA (deoxyribonucleic acid), found mainly in cell nuclei, and RNA (ribonucleic acid), found mostly in cytoplasm. Each nucleic acid chain is composed of subunits called nucleotides, each containing a sugar, a phosphate group, and one of four bases: adenine (symbolized A), guanine (G), cytosine (C) and thymine (T). RNA contains the sugar ribose instead of deoxyribose and the base uracil (U) instead of thymine. The specific sequences of nucleotides constitute the cell's genetic information: Each three-nucleotide DNA sequence specifies one particular amino acid. The long sequences of DNA nucleotides thus correspond to the sequences of amino acids in the cell's proteins. In order to be expressed as protein, the genetic information is carried to the protein-synthesizing machinery of the cell, usually in the cell cytoplasm. Forms of RNA mediate this process. DNA not only provides information, but also specifies its own exact replication. The cell replicates its DNA by making a complementary copy of its exact nucleotide sequence: T for every A, C for every G, G for every C, A for every T. Although the triplet nucleotide code seems to be universal, the actual sequences of the nucleotides vary according to the species and individual. See also Gene; Genetic Engineering; Mutation.

NUCLEOLI: Bodies in the nucleus that become enlarged during protein synthesis and contain the DNA template for ribosomal RNA. See also Ribonucleic Acid; Ribosome.

NUCLEOSIDE ANALOG: Nucleosides are related to nucleotides, the subunits of nucleic acids; however, they do not carry the phosphate groups of the nucleotides. Nucleoside analogs generally are synthetic compounds similar to one of the components of DNA or RNA; a general type of antiviral drug (e.g., acyclovir and AZT). See also Acyclovir; AZT; Nucleic Acid.

NUCLEUS: 1. The central controlling body within a living cell, usually a spherical unit enclosed in a membrane and containing genetic codes for maintaining the life systems of the organism and for issuing commands for growth and reproduction. 2. The nucleus of a cell is an organelle (i.e., a cellular organ) that is essential to such cell functions as reproduction and protein synthesis. It is composed of nuclear sap and a nucleoprotein-rich network from which chromosomes and nucleoli arise and is enclosed in a definite membrane. See also Nucleoli.

OPEN-LABEL TRIAL: A clinical trial in which doctors and participants know which drug or vaccine is being administered. See also Clinical Trial.

OPPORTUNISTIC INFECTION: 1. An illness caused by an organism that usually does not cause disease in a person with a normal immune system. People with advanced HIV infection suffer opportunistic infections of the lungs, brain, eyes and other organs. 2. Opportunistic infections common in AIDS patients include Pneumocystis carinii pneumonia, Kaposi's sarcoma, shigellosis, histoplasmosis and other parasitic, viral, and fungal infections, and some types of cancers. See also Histoplasmosis; Kaposi's Sarcoma; Pneumocystis carinii Pneumonia.

OROPHARYNGEAL: Relating to that division of the pharynx between the soft palate and the epiglottis. Pharynx is a tube that connects the mouth and nasal passages with the esophagus, the connection to the stomach. Epiglottis is a thin, valvelike structure that covers the glottis, the opening of the upper part of the larynx (the part of the throat containing the vocal cords), during swallowing.

PALLIATIVE: A treatment that provides symptomatic relief, but not a cure.

PANCREAS: A gland situated near the stomach that secretes a digestive fluid into the intestine through one or more ducts and also secretes the hormone insulin.

PANCREATITIS: Inflammation of the pancreas that can produce severe pain and debilitating illness. See also Pancreas.

PANCYTOPENIA: Deficiency of all cell elements of the blood.

PANDEMIC: A disease prevalent throughout an entire country, continent or the whole world. See also Epidemic.

PAP SMEAR: A method for the early detection of cancer and other abnormalities of the female genital tract, especially of the cervix and uterus, employing exfoliated cells (cells that have been shed into vaginal fluid) and a special staining technique for microscopic examination that differentiates diseased tissue. Also known as Papanicolaou Smear after George Papanicolaou, the American cytologist who developed this method and published it in 1943. See also Cervix; Uterus.

PAPILLOMA: 1. A benign tumor (as a wart or condyloma) resulting from an overgrowth of epithelial tissue on papillae of vascularized connective tissue (as of the skin). 2. An epithelial tumor caused by a virus. See also Condyloma; Epithelium.

PARALLEL TRACK: A system of distributing experimental drugs to patients who are unable to participate in ongoing clinical efficacy trials and have no other treatment options. See also Clinical Trial.

PARASITE: A plant or animal that lives and feeds on or within another living organism; does not necessarily cause disease.

PARENCHYMA: The tissue of an organ (as distinguished from supporting or connective tissue).

PARENTERAL: Not in or through the digestive system. For example, parenteral can pertain to blood being drawn from a vein in the arm or introduced into that vein via a transfusion (intravenous), or to injection of medications or vaccines through the skin (subcutaneous) or into the muscle (intramuscular).

PARESTHESIA: Any subjective sensation, experienced as numbness, tingling or a "pins-and-needles" feeling.

PATHOGEN: Any disease-producing microorganism or material.

PEER REVIEW: The process by which new scientific or medical findings, announced by one researcher, are reviewed by other scientists or physicians before these findings are published.

PELVIC INFLAMMATORY DISEASE (PID): A term used to describe infections of the uterus, the fallopian tubes and the ovaries. PID is usually the result of untreated sexually transmitted disease, primarily chlamydia or gonorrhea. See also Fallopian Tubes; Ovary; Uterus.

PENTAMIDINE: An approved antiprotozoal drug used for the treatment and prevention of Pneumocystis carinii pneumonia (PCP) infection. It can be delivered intravenously or intramuscularly or inhaled as an aerosol. Aerosolized pentamidine is approved for the prophylaxis of PCP in HIV-positive individuals with CD4+ counts below 200 per cubic millimeter or for those with prior episodes of PCP. The drug is also known under the names Pentam and NebuPent. See also Pneumocystis carinii Pneumonia.

PHAGOCYTE: A cell that is able to ingest and destroy foreign matter, including bacteria.

PHAGOCYTOSIS: The process of ingesting and destroying a virus or other foreign matter by phagocyte. See also Macrophage; Monocyte.

PHARMACOKINETICS: The processes (in a living organism) of absorption, distribution, metabolism and excretion of a drug or vaccine.

PHYTOHEMAGGLUTININ (PHA): A plant chemical used to stimulate the multiplication of white blood cells.

PITUITARY GLAND: Small, oval endocrine gland that lies at the base of the brain. It is called the master gland because the other endocrine glands depend on its secretions for stimulation. The pituitary has two distinct lobes, anterior and posterior. The anterior lobe secretes at least six hormones: human growth hormone, which stimulates overall body growth; ACTH(adrenocorticotropic hormone), which controls steroid hormone secretion by the adrenal cortex; thyrotropic hormone, which stimulates the activity of the thyroid gland; and three gonadotropic hormones, which control growth and reproductive activity of the gonads (ovaries and testes). The posterior lobe secretes antidiuretic hormone, which causes water retention by the kidneys, and oxytocin, which stimulates the mammary glands to release milk and also causes uterine contractions. An overactive pituitary during childhood can cause gigantism; during adulthood, it can cause acromegaly. Dwarfism results from pituitary deficiency in childhood. See also Acromegaly.

PLACEBO: An inactive substance against which investigational treatments are compared for efficacy. See also Placebo Controlled Study.

PLACEBO CONTROLLED STUDY: A method of investigation of drugs in which an inactive substance (the placebo) is given to one group of patients, while the drug being tested is given to another group. The results obtained in the two groups are then compared.

PLACEBO EFFECT: A physical or emotional change occurring after a substance is taken or administered that is not the result of any special property of the substance. The change may be beneficial, reflecting the expectations of the patient and, often, the expectations of the person giving the substance.

PLASMA: That 10 percent of the blood that contains nutrients, electrolytes (dissolved salts), gases, albumin, clotting factors, wastes and hormones.

PLASMA CELLS: Large antibody-producing cells that develop from B cells. See also Antibodies; B Lymphocytes.

PLASMAPHERESIS: The selective removal of certain proteins or antibodies from the blood (followed by reinjection of the blood). This process is sometimes used in the treatment of some peripheral neuropathies and is an integral part of passive immunotherapies for HIV. See also Neuropathy.

PLATELETS: Active agents of inflammation when damage occurs to a blood vessel. They are not actually cells, but fragments released by megakaryocyte cells. Megakaryocyte is a large cell in the bone marrow whose function is to produce platelets. When vascular damage (i.e., damage to blood vessels) occurs, the platelets stick to the vascular walls, forming clots to prevent the loss of blood. Thus, it is important to have adequate numbers of normally functioning platelets to maintain effective coagulation of the blood. There are drugs that can potentially alter the platelet count, making it necessary to monitor the count. Also, some people with HIV infection develop thrombocytopenia (a condition characterized by a platelet count of less than 100,000 platelets per cubic millimeter of blood). The normal value for men is 154,000-354,000 platelets per cubic millimeter of blood. For women, it is 162,000-380,000 platelets per cubic millimeter of blood.

PNEUMOCYSTIS CARINII PNEUMONIA (PCP): 1. A protozoal infection of the lungs. 2. A life-threatening lung infection that can affect people with weakened immune systems, such as those infected with HIV. More than three-quarters of all people with HIV disease will develop PCP if they do not receive treatment to prevent it. The standard treatment for people with PCP is either a combination of trimethoprim and sulfamethoxazole.

POLYMERASE: Any of several enzymes that catalyze the formation of DNA or RNA from precursor substances in the presence of preexisting DNA or RNA acting as templates (i.e., patterns).

POLYMERASE CHAIN REACTION (PCR): 1. A laboratory process that selects a DNA segment from a mixture of

DNA chains and rapidly replicates it; used to create a large, readily analyzed sample of a piece of DNA. It is used in DNA fingerprinting and in medical tests to identify diseases from the infectious agent's DNA. See also DNA. 2. As related to HIV: A sensitive laboratory technique that can detect and quantify HIV in a person's blood or lymph node.

POLYVALENT VACCINE: A vaccine that is active against multiple viral strains.

PRECURSOR CELLS: Cells from which other cells are formed by natural processes.

PREVALENCE: A measure of the proportion of people in a population affected with a particular disease at a given time.

PROPHYLAXIS: Treatment that helps to prevent a disease or condition before it occurs or recurs.

PROTEASE: An enzyme that hydrolyzes (i.e., breaks down) proteins to their component peptides. See also Enzyme; Peptide; Proteins.

PROTEASE INHIBITORS: HIV protease is an aspartyl enzyme essential to the replicative life cycle of HIV. The three-dimensional molecular structure of the HIV protease has been fully determined. Pharmaceutical developers are therefore able to rationally design compounds to inhibit it and thus interfere with replication of the virus. In the US, five peptide-based protease inhibitors (saquinavir, Roche; A-80987, ABT-538, Abbott Laboratories; L735,524, Merck; KNI-272, NCI) are in clinical development. All compounds inhibit HIV-1 in vitro in nanomolar concentrations. In Europe, two peptide-based compounds (ABT-987, Abbott Laboratories; AG-1343, Agouron Pharmaceuticals, Inc.) are currently in development. See also In Vitro.

PROTEINS: Any of the group of highly complex organic compounds found in all living cells. Protein is the most abundant class of all biological molecules, comprising about 50 percent of cellular dry weight. Classified by biological function, proteins include the enzymes, which catalyze cellular reactions; collagen, keratin and elastin, which are structural, or support, proteins; hemoglobin and other transport proteins; casein, ovalbumin and other nutrient proteins; antibodies, which are necessary for immunity; protein hormones, which regulate metabolism; and proteins such as actin and myosin, the contractile muscle proteins that perform mechanical work. Structurally, proteins are large molecules composed of one or more chains of varying amounts of the same 22 amino acids, which are linked by peptide bonds. Each protein is characterized by a unique and invariant amino acid sequence. Protein chains may contain hundreds of amino acids; some proteins also incorporate phosphorus or such metals as iron, zinc and copper. The amino acid sequence also determines the molecule's three-dimensional structure; this so-called native state is required for proper biological function. The information for the syntheses of the specific amino acid sequences from free amino acids is carried by the cell's nucleic acid. See also Peptide; Ribonucleic Acid.

PROTOCOL: The detailed plan for a clinical trial that states the trial's rationale, purpose, drug or vaccine dosages, length of study, routes of administration, who may participate and other aspects of trial design. See also Clinical Trial; Inclusion/Exclusion Criteria.

PROTOPLASM: Fundamental material composing all living things. Protoplasm, which exists in all plants and animals in the small units called cells, is mainly (85-90 percent) water and also contains proteins, fatty substances and inorganic salts. It is always enclosed by a thin surface membrane that controls the passage of materials into and out of the cell. It displays the general properties associated with life-the capacity to respond to stimuli and the ability to perform the essential physiological functions.

PUBLIC HEALTH SERVICE (PHS): A multi-agency organizational component of the US Department of Health and Human Services. See also Centers for Disease Control and Prevention; Health Resources and Services Administration; National Institutes of Health.

REACTOGENICITY: The capacity to produce adverse reactions.

RECEPTOR: A molecule on the surface of a cell that serves as a recognition or binding site for antigens, antibodies or other cellular or immunological components.

RECOMBINANT: An organism whose genome contains integrated genetic material from a different organism. See also Genome.

REGULATORY GENES: As related to HIV: Three regulatory HIV genes-tat, rev and nef-and three so-called auxiliary genes-vif, vpr and vpu-contain information for the production of proteins that control (i.e., regulate) the virus's ability to infect a cell, produce new copies of the virus or cause disease. See also nef; rev; tat.

REGULATORY T CELLS: T cells that direct other immune cells to perform special functions. The chief regulatory cell, the CD4+ T cell or T helper cell, is HIV's chief target. See also CD4 (T4) or CD4+ Cells; T Cells.

REMISSIONS: The lessening of the severity or duration of outbreaks of a disease, or the abatement (diminution in degree or intensity) of symptoms altogether over a period of time.

RETICULOENDOTHELIAL CELLS: A system of interstitial cells that includes all the phagocytic cells, which trap and consume foreign agents, except the leukocytes circulating in the bloodstream. This system forms a network throughout the body and is another of the body's defense systems against invading organisms in the connective tissues of the body. See also Leukocytes; Phagocyte.

RETINA: Light-sensitive tissue at the back of the eye that transmits visual impulses via the optic nerve to the brain.

RETINITIS: Inflammation of the retina, linked in AIDS to CMV infection. Untreated, it can lead to blindness. See also Cytomegalovirus; Retina.

RETROVIRUS: HIV and other viruses that carry their genetic material in the form of RNA and that have the enzyme reverse transcriptase. Like all viruses, HIV can replicate only inside cells, commandeering the cell's machinery to reproduce. Like other retroviruses, HIV uses the enzyme called reverse transcriptase to convert its RNA into DNA, which is then integrated into the host cell DNA. See also DNA; Reverse Transcriptase; Ribonucleic Acid.

REV: One of the regulatory genes of the HIV virus. Three HIV regulatory genes-tat, rev and nef-and three so-called auxiliary genes-vif, vpr and vpu-contain information necessary for the production of proteins that control the virus's ability to infect a cell, produce new copies of the virus or cause disease. See also nef; tat.

REVERSE TRANSCRIPTASE: This enzyme of the HIV virus (and other retroviruses) converts the single-stranded viral RNA into DNA, the form in which the cell carries its genes. The antiviral drugs approved in the US for the treatment of HIV infection-AZT, ddC and ddI-all work by interfering with this stage of the viral life cycle. See also AZT; ddC; ddI; DNA; Ribonucleic Acid.

RIBONUCLEIC ACID (RNA): 1. A nucleic acid, found mostly in the cytoplasm of cells, that is important in the synthesis of proteins. The amount of RNA varies from cell to cell. RNA, like the structurally similar DNA, is a chain made up of subunits called nucleotides. In protein synthesis, messenger RNA (mRNA) replicates the DNA code for a protein and moves to sites in the cell called ribosomes. There, transfer RNA (tRNA) assembles amino acids to form the protein specified by the messenger RNA. Most forms of RNA (including messenger and transfer RNA) consist of a single nucleotide strand, but a few forms of viral RNA that function as carriers of genetic information (instead of DNA) are double-stranded. 2. A nucleic acid associated with the control of chemical activities inside a cell. One type of RNA transfers information from the cell's DNA to the protein-forming system of a cell outside the nucleus. Some viruses (e.g., HIV) carry RNA instead of the more usual genetic material DNA. See also Cytoplasm; DNA; Retrovirus.

RIBOSOME: A cytoplasmic organelle composed of ribonucleic acid and protein that functions in the synthesis of protein. Ribosomes interact with messenger RNA and transfer RNA to join together amino acid units into a polypeptide chain according to the sequence determined by the genetic code. See also Cytoplasm; Ribonucleic Acid.

SEROCONVERSION: The development of antibodies to a particular antigen. When people develop antibodies to HIV or an experimental HIV vaccine, they "seroconvert" from antibody-negative to antibody-positive. See also Antibodies; Antigen.

SEROPREVALENCE: As related to HIV infection: The proportion of persons who have serologic (i.e., pertaining to serum) evidence of HIV infection at any given time. See also Serum.

SEROSTATUS: Results of a test for specific antibodies. See also Antibodies.

SERUM: The clear, thin and sticky fluid portion of the blood that remains after coagulation. Serum contains no blood cells, platelets or fibrinogen.

SEXUALLY TRANSMITTED DISEASE (STD): Also called venereal disease. A contagious disease usually acquired by sexual intercourse or genital contact. Historically, the five venereal diseases were: gonorrhea, syphilis, chancroid, granuloma inguinale and lymphogranuloma venereum. To these have been added scabies, herpes genitalis and anorectal herpes and warts, pediculosis, trichomoniasis, genital candidiasis, molluscum contagiosum, nonspecific urethritis, chlamydial infections, cytomegalovirus and AIDS. See also Herpes Simplex Virus II; Molluscum Contagiosum.

SHIV: Genetically engineered hybrid virus having an HIV envelope and an SIV core. See also Genetic Engineering; Hybrid; Simian Immunodeficiency Virus.

SIDE EFFECTS: The action or effect of a drug (or vaccine) other than that desired. The term usually refers to undesired or negative effects, such as headache, skin irritation or liver damage. Experimental drugs must be evaluated for both immediate and long-term side effects.

SIMIAN IMMUNODEFICIENCY VIRUS (SIV): An HIV-like virus that infects monkeys, chimpanzees and other nonhuman primates.

STANDARDS OF CARE: Treatment regimen or medical management based on state-of-the-art patient care.

STATISTICAL SIGNIFICANCE: A term based on statistical tests that is used to denote the probability that the observed association could have occurred by chance alone. Does not refer to medical or biological significance of an association. For example, a statistical significance at the 1-percent level indicates a 1-in-100 chance that a result can be ascribed to chance.

STEM CELLS: Cells from which all blood cells derive. Bone marrow is rich in stem cells.

STERILIZING IMMUNITY: An immune response that completely eliminates an infection.

STEVENS-JOHNSON SYNDROME: A severe and sometimes fatal form of erythema multiforme that is characterized by conjunctivitis (eye inflammation) and often results in blindness, Vincent's angina (trench mouth) and ulceration of the genitals and anus. See also Erythema Multiforme.

STOMATITIS: Any of numerous inflammatory diseases of the mouth having various causes, such as mechanical trauma, irritants, allergy, vitamin deficiency or infection.

SUBUNIT HIV VACCINE: A genetically engineered vaccine that is based on only part of the HIV molecule. See also Genetic Engineering.

SULFA DRUG: Any of a class of synthetic chemical substances derived from sulfanilamide and used to treat bacterial infections. These drugs inhibit the action of para-aminobenzoic acid, a substance bacteria needed in order to reproduce. Sulfa drugs are used primarily in the treatment of urinary tract infections and ulcerative colitis. Antibiotics have largely replaced them in the treatment of other bacterial infections.

SUPERANTIGEN: Investigators have proposed that a molecule known as a superantigen, either made by HIV or an unrelated agent, may stimulate massive quantities of CD4+ T cells at once, rendering them highly susceptible to HIV infection and subsequent cell death. See also Antigen; CD4 (T4) or CD4+ Cells.

SURROGATE MARKER: A substitute; a person or thing that replaces another. In HIV disease, the number of CD4+ T cells and CD8+ cells is a surrogate immunological marker of disease progression. See also CD4 (T4) or CD4+ Cells; CD8 (T8) Cells.

SURVEILLANCE: Close or continuous observation or testing (e.g., serosurveillance), used, among others, in epidemiology. Immunological surveillance, or immunosurveillance, is a monitoring process of the immune system that detects and destroys neoplastic (e.g., cancerous) cells and that tends to break down in immunosuppressed individuals. See also Epidemiologic Surveillance.

SUSCEPTIBLE: Vulnerable or predisposed to a disease.

SYMPTOMS: Any perceptible, subjective change in the body or its functions that indicates disease or phases of disease, as reported by the patient.

SYNCYTIA: ("Giant Cells"). Dysfunctional multicellular clumps formed by cell-to-cell fusion. Cells infected with HIV may also fuse with nearby uninfected cells, forming balloonlike giant cells called syncytia. In test tube experiments, these giant cells have been associated with the death of uninfected cells. The presence of so-called syncytia-inducing variants of HIV has been correlated with rapid disease progression in HIV-infected individuals.

SYNDROME: A group of symptoms and diseases that together are characteristic of a specific condition.

SYNERGISM/SYNERGISTIC: An interaction between two or more agents (drugs) that produces or enhances an effect that is greater than the sum of the effects produced by the individual agents.

SYNTHESIS: 1. In chemistry, the formation of a compound from simpler compounds or elements. 2. The production of a substance (e.g., as in protein synthesis) by the union of chemical elements, groups or simpler compounds, or by the degradation (i.e., breaking down) of a complex compound.

T CELLS: (T Lymphocytes). A thymus-derived white blood cell that participates in a variety of cell-mediated immune reactions. Three fundamentally different types of T cells are recognized: helper, killer and suppressor (each has many subdivisions). T lymphocytes are CD3+ and can be separated into the CD4+ T helper cells and the CD8+ cytotoxic/suppresssor cells. See also Thymus.

TEMPLATE: A gauge, pattern or mold used as a guide to the form of the piece being made. In biology, a molecule (such as DNA) that serves as a pattern for the generation of another macromolecule (e.g., messenger RNA).

TERATOGENICITY: The production of physical defects in offspring in utero (i.e., causing birth defects).

THERAPEUTIC HIV VACCINE: A vaccine designed to boost the immune response to HIV in persons already infected with the virus.

3TC: Also known as Lamivudine, 3TC is composed of the (-) enantiomer of the racemic mixture 2'-deoxy-3'-thiacytidine. Like other nucleoside analogs, 3TC inhibits HIV replication through viral DNA chain termination. It has been used in clinical trials in combination with AZT. See also AZT; Nucleoside Analog.

THROMBOCYTOPENIA: A decreased number of blood platelets (cells important for blood clotting). See also Platelets.

THRUSH: Sore patches in the mouth caused by the fungus Candida albicans. Thrush is one of the most frequent early symptoms of an immune disorder. The fungus commonly lives in the mouth, but only causes problems when the body's resistance is reduced either by antibiotics that have reduced the number of competitive organisms in the mouth, or by an immune deficiency such as HIV disease. See also Candida.

THYMOSIN: A polypeptide hormone of the thymus that influences the maturation of T cells destined for an active role in cell-mediated immunity. See also T Cells; Thymus.

THYMUS: A mass of glandular tissue located in the neck or chest of most vertebrates. Found in the upper chest under the breastbone in humans, the thymus is essential to the development of the body's system of immunity beginning in fetal life (i.e., before birth). The thymus processes white blood cells, known as lymphocytes, which kill foreign cells and stimulate other immune cells to produce antibodies. The gland grows throughout childhood until puberty and then gradually decreases in size. See also Antibodies; Lymphocyte.

TISSUE: A collection of similar cells acting together to perform a particular function. There are four basic tissues in the body: epithelial, connective, muscle and nerve.

TITER: (Also "titre"). A laboratory measurement of the amount (or concentration) of a given compound in solution.

T LYMPHOCYTE PROLIFERATION ASSAY: Measures the strength of response of T memory cells (a subgroup of T lymphocytes) to HIV. See also T Cells.

TOXICITY: The extent, quality or degree of being poisonous or harmful to the body.

TOXOPLASMOSIS: Toxoplasmosis is an infection that is caused by the protozoan parasite Toxoplasma gondii. The parasite is carried by cats, birds and other animals and is found in soil contaminated by cat feces and in meat, particularly pork. The parasite can infect the lungs, retina of the eye, heart, pancreas, liver, colon and testes. Once T. gondii invades the body, it remains there, but the immune system in a healthy person usually prevents the parasite from causing disease. If the immune system becomes severely damaged, as in people with AIDS, or is suppressed by drugs, T. gondii can begin to multiply and cause severe disease. The most common site of toxoplasmosis is the brain. When T. gondii invades the brain, causing inflammation, the condition is called toxoplasmic encephalitis. While the disease can occur in persons with healthy immune systems, it can normally be cured successfully. See also Protozoa.

TRANSCRIPTION: The process of constructing a messenger RNA molecule using a DNA molecule as a template with the resulting transfer of genetic information to the messenger RNA. As related to HIV: The process by which the provirus produces new viruses. RNA copies called messenger RNA must be made that can be read by the host cell's protein-making machinery. Transcription is facilitated by cellular enzymes, including RNA polymerase

II. The viral genes may partly control this process: tat, for example, encodes a protein that accelerates the transcription process by binding to a section of the newly made viral RNA. See also Integration; Messenger RNA; tat; Template.

TRANSFER FACTOR: A fraction of white blood cells that apparently "transfers" capability to mount an immune response to a specific antigen. See also Antigen.

TRANSFUSION: 1. The process of transfusing fluid (such as blood) into a vein. 2. The transfer of whole blood or blood products from one individual to another.

TRANSLATION: As related to HIV: The process by which HIV messenger RNA is processed in a cell's nucleus and transported to the cytoplasm, the cellular material outside the nucleus. In the cytoplasm, the cell's protein-making machinery translates the messenger RNA into viral protein and enzymes. See also Cytoplasm; Enzyme; Messenger RNA; Nucleus.

TRANSMISSION: In the context of HIV disease: HIV is spread most commonly by sexual contact with an infected partner. The virus can enter the body through the mucosal lining of the vagina, vulva, penis, rectum or, very rarely, the mouth during sex. The likelihood of transmission is increased by factors that may damage these linings, especially other sexually transmitted diseases that cause ulcers or inflammation. Studies of SIV infection of the genital membranes of nonhuman primates suggest that the sentinel cells known as mucosal dendritic cells may be the first cells infected. Infected dendritic cells may migrate to lymph nodes and infect other cells. HIV also is spread through contact with infected blood, most often by the sharing of drug needles or syringes contaminated with minute quantities of blood containing the virus. Children can contract HIV from their infected mothers either during pregnancy or birth, or postnatally, via breastfeeding. Current research indicates that the AIDS virus may be 100 to 1000 times more contagious during the first two months of infection, when routine AIDS tests are unable to tell whether people are infected. See also Lymph Nodes; Simian Immunodeficiency Virus.

TREATMENT IND: A program to provide experimental treatments to a class of patients who lack satisfactory alternative treatment. IND stands for Investigational New Drug application, which is part of the process to get approval from the Food and Drug Administration for marketing a new prescription drug in the US. See also Investigational New Drug.

UTERUS: A hollow muscular organ located in the pelvic cavity of female mammals in which the fertilized egg implants and develops. Also called womb.

VACCINATION: Inoculation of a substance (vaccine) into the body for the purpose of producing active immunity against a disease. The vaccine is usually a weakened culture of the agent causing the disease; the use of vaccines is a cornerstone of preventive medicine. Vaccination was used in ancient times in China, India and Persia, and was introduced to the West in the late 18th century by E. Jenner. Vaccinations have eradicated smallpox and are used today to prevent diphtheria, poliomyelitis, rabies and typhoid. Experimental vaccines for certain cancers have been developed for laboratory mice.

VACCINE: A substance that contains antigenic components from an infectious organism. By stimulating an immune response (but not disease), it protects against subsequent infection by that organism. See also Antigen; Vaccination.

VACCINIA: A cowpox virus, formerly used in human smallpox vaccines. Employed as a vector in HIV vaccine research to transport HIV genes into the body. See also Vaccination; Vector.

VARIABLE REGION: The part of an antibody's structure

that differs from one antibody to another. See also Antibodies.

VECTOR: A nonpathogenic bacterium or virus used to transport an antigen into the body to stimulate protective immunity (e.g., in a vaccine). See also Antigen.

VIRAL BURDEN: (Viral Load). The amount of HIV virus in the circulating blood. Monitoring a person's viral burden is important because of the apparent correlation between the amount of virus in the blood and the severity of the disease: sicker patients generally have more virus than those with less advanced disease. A new, sensitive, rapid test-called the branched DNA assay for HIV-1 infection-can be used to monitor the HIV viral burden. In the future, this procedure may help clinicians to decide when to give anti-HIV therapy. It may also help investigators determine more quickly if experimental HIV therapies are effective.

VIRAL ENVELOPE: As related to HIV: HIV is spherical in shape with a diameter of 1/10,000 of a millimeter. The outer coat, or envelope, is composed of two layers of fat-like molecules called lipids, taken from the membranes of human cells. Embedded in the envelope are numerous cellular proteins, as well as mushroom-shaped HIV proteins that protrude from the surface. Each mushroom is thought toconsist of a cap made of four glycoprotein molecules called gp120, and a stem consisting of four gp41 molecules embedded in the envelope. The virus uses these proteins to attach to and infect cells.

Bibliography

Albury, Rebecca. (1990). Sexual Politics in the 1990s: Making Sex Safer?. Social Alternatives, 9(1).

Alexander, Nancy J. et.al. (1990). Heterosexual Transmissi n of AIDS. New York: Wiley.Altman, D., *Power and Commun ty: Organisational and Cultural* Responses *to AIDS*. London: Taylor and

Francis, 1994.

Anastos, Kathryn and Marte, Carola. (1991). Women - The Missing Persons in the AIDS Epidemic. In McKenzie, Nancy F. (ed.). The AIDS Reader: Social, Political, and Ethical Issues. New York: Meridian.

Anderson, Jean R., ed. *A Guide to the Clinical Care of Women with HIV/AIDS*. Rockville, Md, 2001.

Barnett T., and Whiteside A., *AIDS in the Twenty-First Century*. Chippenham and Eastbourne. Antony Rowe Ltd., 2002.

Boulton, Mary, Evans, Zoe S., Fitzpatrick, Ray and Hart, Graham. (1991). Bisexual Men: Women, Safer Sex and HIV Transmission. In Aggleton, Peter, Hart, Graham and Davies, Peter. (eds). AIDS: Responses, Interventions and Care. London: Falmer Press.

Bourdieu, P. and J.C. Passeron, 1977, *Reproduction in Education. Society and Culture.* London: Sage.

Census of India 1981a Series 11, Madhya Pradesh, Part

11-A. General Population Tables Controller of Publications, New Delhi.

Census of India 1981b Series 11, Madhya Pradesh, Part 11, Special Reports and Tables Based on 5 Per cent Sample Data. Controller of Publications, New Delhi.

Census of India 1981d Series 1, India, Paper 1 of 1984. Population Projections for India 1981-2001. Controller of Publications, New Delhi.

Chen, Lincoln C., J.S. Amor, and Sheldon J. Segal. (1992). AIDS and Women's Reproductive Health. New York: Plenum Publishing Corporation.

Clatts, Michael C. and Payne, Kenneth. (1989). AIDS and the Dangerous Other: Metaphors of Sex and Deviance in the Representation of Disease. In Bolton, Ralph. (ed.). The AIDS Pandemic: A Global Emergency. New York: Gordon and Breach.

Clayman, Charles B., (Ed.). *The American Medical Association Encyclopedia of Medicine*, Random House, New York, 1991.

Cline, Rebecca J. Welch and McKenzie, Nelya J. (1994). Sex Differences in Communication and the Construction of HIV/AIDS. Journal of Applied Communication Research, 22, 4, November, pp. 322-337.

Cochran, Susan D. and Mays, Vickie M. (1990). Sex, Lies and HIV. New England Journal of Medicine, March 15, 322, pp. 774-5.

Cochran, Susan D. and Peplau, Letitia, Anne P. (1991). Sexual Risk Reduction Behaviours Among Young Heterosexual Adults. Social Science and Medicine, 33(1).

Cochrane Collaboration. *Research glossary for consumers.* 1999. Available on line at: www.cochrane.org/cochrane/cngloss.htm.

Cohen, Cathy J. (1996). Contested Membership: Black Gay Identities and the Politics of AIDS. In Seidman, Steven. (ed). (1996). Queer Theory/Sociology. Cambridge, Ma: Blackwell).

Cohen, D., *Mainstreaming the policy and programming response to the HIV epidemic,* New York, UNDP. 2000.

Cohen, Felissa L. and Durham, Jerry D. (eds). (1993). Women, Children and HIV/AIDS. New York: Springer.

Cohen, Felissa L., Epidemiology of HIV Infection and AIDS in Adolescents, *Women, Children and HIV/AIDS*, Springer Publishing, New York, 1993.

Columbia University College of Physicians and Surgeons, *Complete Home Medical Guide*, Columbia University Press, New York, 1989.

Community Research Initiative of Toronto (CRIT), Canadian HIV Trials Network (CTN) - Ontario Region, HIV Ontario Observational Database (HOOD). *A workbook for community-based research.* Toronto: CRIT, CTN, HOOD, 1996.

Connell, R.W. and Kippax, Susan. (1990). Sexuality in the AIDS Crisis: Patterns of Sexual Practice and Pleasure in a Sample of Australian Gay and Bisexual Men. Journal of Sex Research, 27(2).

Connell, R.W., Crawford, J., Dowsett, G.W., Kippax, S., Sinnott, V., Baxter, D. and Watson, L. (1990). Danger and Context: Unsafe Anal Sexual Practice Among Homosexual and Bisexual Men in the AIDS Crisis. Australian and New Zealand Journal of Sociology, 26(2), August.

Connell, R.W., Crawford, J., Kippax, S., Dowsett, G.W., Baxter, D., Watson, L. and Berg, R. (1989). Facing the Epidemic: Changes in the Sexual Lives of Gay and

Bisexual Men in Australia and Their Implications for AIDS Prevention Strategies. Social Problems, 36(4).

Coombe, C. Kelly M., "Education as a vehicle for combating HIV/AIDS", *UNESCO Prospects:* 31(3): 435-445), 2001.

Coombe, C., *Managing the impact of HIV/AIDS on the education sector,* University of Pretoria: Centre for the study of AIDS. 2000.

Corbett, E.L., Watt, C.J., Walker. N., et al., "The growing burden of tuberculosis: global trends and interactions with the HIV epidemic", *Archives of Internal Medicine,* 163:100-921, 2003.

Corbett. E.L., Watt, C.J., Walker, N., et al., "The growing burden of tuberculosis: global trends and interactions with the HIV epidemic". *Archives of Internal Medicine.* 163:100-921. 2003.

Coxon, Anthony et.al. (1993). Research Note: Strategies in Eliciting Sensitive Sexual Information: The Case of Gay Men. Sociological Review, 41(3), August.

Crimp, Douglas. (2002). Melancholia and Moralism: Essays on AIDS and queer politics. Cambridge, Mass.: MIT Press.

Crimp, Douglas. (ed). (1988). AIDS: Cultural Analysis/ Cultural Activism. Cambridge and London: MIT Press (Originally published as "AIDS: Cultural Analysis/ Cultural Activism". October 43, Winter 1987).

Crofts N., et al. "Harm Reduction in Asia: A successful response to hidden epidemics", *AIDS:* 12 (supplement B): S109-S115. 1998.

Crossley, Michele L. (2001). How to use a condom: Narratives, sexualities and moralities in safer sex health promotional literature. Culture, Health & Sexuality, Volume 3 Number 3, July, pp. 363-370.

Desmond C., Michael K, Gow J., *The Hidden Battle:* HIV/AIDS in the *Family and Community,* Health Economics and HIV-AID Research Division (HEARD). Durban: University of Natal, 2001.

Development in India", Background Study for the Swedish Country Strategy for India 2003-2007, Sida, New Delhi. 2003.

DFW, 1987, *The Methodology of Setting Targets for Family Planning Programme --A Resume,* circulated by Department of Family Welfare, Ministry of Health and Family Welfare, Government of India Delhi

Dharma Vira, "Citizen Participation" in *Encyclopaedia of Social Work,* Vol. I, p. 102.

Dorn, Nicholas, Henderson, Sheila and South, Nigel. (eds). (1992). AIDS: Women, Drugs and Social Care. London and Washington D.C.: Falmer Press.

Dowsett, Gary W. (1990). Reaching Men Who Have Sex With Men in Australia. An Overview of AIDS Education: Community Intervention and Community Attachment Strategies. Australian Journal of Social Issues, 25(3).

Dowsett, Gary W. (1992a). Practising Desire: Homosexual Sex in the Era of AIDS. PhD thesis, Sociology, School of Behavioural Sciences, Macquarie University. Sydney.

Dowsett, Gary W. (1992b). The Sociological Context. In Timewell, Eric, Minichiello, Victor and Plummer, David. (eds). AIDS in Australia, Parramatta, NSW: Prentice Hall.

Food and Agriculture Organization. *Living Well with HIV/AIDS: A Manual on Nutritional Care and Support for People Living with HIV/AIDS.* Geneva, 2002.

Francis-Xavier Bagnoud Center, UMDNJ, Health Resources and Services Administration and the National Institutes of Health. *Guidelines for the Use of Antiretroviral Agents in Pediatric HIV Infection.* January 20, 2004.

Furler M, Walmsley S, Millson P et al. *Antiretroviral medication use by Ontario HIV patients: gender differences.* Canadian Journal of Infectious Diseases 2001;12 Suppl B:72B.

Gillespie, A., Birdthistle, I., Jones, J., Bundy, D.A.P., Hoffman, AM., Pigozzi, M., Draxler, A., Vince Whitman, C., Fouilhoux, M., Drake, L. (2003). Focusing Resources on Effective School Health: A FRESH start to enhancing HIV/AIDS prevention. Commonwealth Education Partnerships, 2003.pp 80-84.

Gilmore, N. and M.A. Somerville, "Stigmatisation, scapegoating and discrimination in sexually transmitted diseases, overcoming 'them' and 'us'," *Social Science and Medicine.* 39:1339-1358. 1994.

Godin, Gaston, Helene Gagnon, and Leo-Daniel Lambert (2003) Factors Associated with Maintenance of Regular Condom Use Among Single Heterosexual Adults. Canadian Journal of Public Health, July / August, 94(4).

Gold, R. S. and Skinner, M. J. (1992). Situational Factors and Thought Processes Associated with Unprotected Intercourse in Young Gay Men. AIDS, 6(9), 1021-1030\.

Gold, R.S., Karmiloff-Smith, A., Skinner, M.J. and Morton, J. (1992). Situational Factors and Thought Processes Associated with Unprotected Intercourse in Heterosexual Students. AIDS Care, 4(3).

Goldstein, Donna M. (1994). AIDS and Women in Brazil: The Emerging Problem. Social Science and Medicine, 39(7).

Goldstein, Nancy and Manlowe, Jennifer L. (eds). (1997).

The Gender Politics of HIV/AIDS in Women: Perspectives on the Pandemic in the United States. New York University Press.

Goldstein, Nancy. (1995). Lesbians and the Medical Profession: HIV/AIDS and the Pursuit of Visibility. Women's Studies, Vol. 24.

Gollub, E.L. and Stein, Z.A. (1993). The New Female Condom: Item 1 on a Women's AIDS Prevention Agenda. American Journal of Public Health, 83(4).

Gorna, Robin. (1996). Vamps, Virgins and Victims: How Can Women fight AIDS?. London & New York: Cassell.

Gostin, L.O. and Z. Lazzarini, *Human Rights and Public Health in the AIDS Pandemic,* New York: Oxford University Press. 1997.

Greene, Warner C., "AIDS and the Immune System," *Scientific American*, September 1993.

Griffin, Gabriele. (1995). Safe and Sexy? Lesbian Erotica in the Age of AIDS. In Pearce, Lynne and Stacey, Jackie. (eds). Romance Revisited. London: Lawrence and Wishart.

Grosskurth H et al.. "Control of sexually transmitted diseases for HIV prevention: understanding the implications of the Mwanza and Rakai trials". *The Lancet.* 2000.

Henderson, Marion, Daniel Wight, Gillian Raab, Charles Abraham, Katie Buston, Graham Hart, and Sue Scott. (2002). Heterosexual risk behaviour among young teenagers in Scotland. Journal of Adolescence, Volume 25, Number 5, October, pp. 483-494.

Hennekens CH, Buring JE. *Epidemiology in medicine.* Boston: Little Brown and Company, 1987.

Herek, Gregory M. and Greene, Beverly. (eds). AIDS, Identity and Community: The HIV Epidemic and Lesbians and Gay Men.

Herold, E.S. and Mewhinney, D.M.K. (1993). Gender Differences in Casual Sex and AIDS Prevention: A Survey of Dating Bars. Journal of Sex Research, 30(1).

Hillier, Lynn, Harrison, Lyn and Warr, Deborah. (1998). When You Carry Condoms all the Boys Think You Want It': Negotiating Competing Discourses about Safe Sex. Journal of Adolescence, 21(1), February.

Hira S.K., Rao Arni SRS, Thaneke J. (1999), Evidence of significant AIDS related mortality in Mumbai Lancet; 354 (9185), pp. 1175-6.

HIV/AIDS Treatment Information Service. *Glossary of HIV/ AIDS related terms*, 3rd ed. Rockville: HIV/AIDS Treatment Information Service, 1999.

Jones and Bartlett, *The Biology of AIDS*, Fan Hang, Boston, 1989.

Jones, Judith. (1991). Young Women and Sexual Health. National AIDS Bulletin, July.

King, Edward. (1993). Safety in Numbers: Safe Sex and Gay Men. London: Cassell.

Leiner, Marvin. (1993). Sexual Politics in Cuba: Machismo, Homosexuality, and AIDS. Westview Press.

Mann, J., D.J.M. Tarantola. and T.W. Netter (ed.), *AIDS in the World*. Boston. MA: Harvard University Press, 1992.

Martindale S, Craib KJ P, Chan K et al. *Increasing rate of new HIV infections among young gay and bisexual men in Vancouver, 1995-99 vs. 2000*. Canadian Journal of Infectious Diseases 2001;12 Suppl B:62B.

Massiah, Hope. (1992). Thinking about the Issues. In

O'Sullivan, Sue and Thomson, Kate. (eds). Positively Women: Living With AIDS. London: Sheba Feminist Press.

Moore, Susan and Rosenthal, Doreen. (1991b). Condoms and Coitus: Adolescents' Attitudes to AIDS and Safe Sex Behaviour. Journal of Adolescence, 14.

Osborn CE. *Statistical applications for health information management.* Gaithersburg, MD: Aspen Publishers, 2000.

Polit DF, Hungler BP. *Essentials of nursing research: methods, appraisal and utilization*, 3rd ed. Philadelphia: J.B. Lippincott, 1993.

Pollack, Michael. (1993). The Second Plague: AIDS Prevention and Sexual Transmission Among Men in Western Europe. New York: Hayworth.

Population, Poverty and the Future of India, by Dr. Karan Singh, p. 89 (Quoted from his speech as "Investment in Man", National Institute of Family Planning, Now Delhi, September 1975.

Rofes, Eric. (1996). Reviving the Tribe: Regenerating Gay Men's Sexuality and Culture in the Ongoing Epidemic. New York & London: Haworth Press.

Rollins, Bruce. (1989). Sexual Attitudes and Behaviours: A Review of the Literature. Melbourne: Australian Institute of Family Studies.

Rosenstock, I.M. 1960: "What Research in Motivation Suggest for Public Health". *American Jour, of Public Health,* 50:295-302.

Rosenthal, Doreen A. (1994). Heterosexuality and HIV/ AIDS. Paper to Harmed Circles: Cultural Responses to the AIDS Crisis, National Gallery of Australia, Canberra, 11-12 November.

Rosenthal, Doreen A., Madeline Fernbach, and Susan M.Moore. (1997). The Singles Scene: Safe Sex Practices and Attitudes Among At-Risk Heterosexual Adults. Psychology and Health, 12.

Saalfield, Catherine and Navarro, Ray. (1991). Shocking Pink Praxis: Race and Gender on the ACT UP Frontlines. In Fuss, Diana. (ed.). Inside/Out: Lesbian Theories, Gay Theories. New York/London: Routledge.

Safety in the Elementary Science Classroom, National Science Teachers Association, Washington, 1978.

Salama, P., Dondero, T., "HIV surveillance in complex emergencies" *AIDS;* 15(3): S4-12.

Singer, Linda. (1993). Erotic Welfare: Sexual Theory and Politics in the Age of Epidemic. New York: Routledge.

Weber AE, Roy E, Blais L et al. *HIV risk and prostitution among females in the Montreal Street Youth Cohort.* Canadian Journal of Infectious Diseases 2001;12 Suppl B:67B.

Index

■■■